"It is her tactics on behalf of disgruntled patients, and her insistence that consumers have a right to know whether their doctor is on probation for drugs or alcohol, or is facing numerous malpractice suits, that has caused unease among . . . physicians." —*The Fresno Bee*

"I could not have enjoyed the book as much as I did had I not met the sensitive, basically shy woman who was forced, against her nature, to become an advocate."
—Joe Stern, Senator, California Senior Legislature

"Thank you for standing tall against the very tremendous and horrible obstacle of medical incompetence."
—Jeanne Rider, Division Chairman, Beta Sigma Phi

" . . . compelling . . . One can appreciate Carroll's approach and her message throughout the book, that people should do things for themselves and not be so quick to hand over responsibilities to 'experts'."
—*Vegetarian Times*

" . . . a tone and style which challenges without stridency, which draws attention without libeling, which touches at heart-level the very institutions and people who have most to lose in the message."
—Paula D'Arpino

" . . . a rare and wonderful woman . . . a thundering message . . . the impact of *Life Wish* is bound to be far-reaching."
—Jayne Murdock in *SPEX*

"This book *reveals* much that all consumers need to know—and hopefully many doctors will also read it. Congratulations on a well written and documented book . . ."
—Vencil T. Ward, Senator, California Senior Legislature

"Congratulations to Paula Carroll and people like her who are trying to wake up the American medical establishment."
—Dana Ullman, M.P.H.

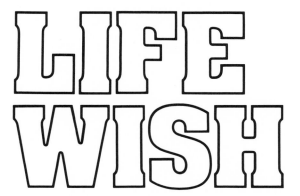

LIFE WISH

One Woman's Struggle
Against Medical Incompetence

PAULA CARROLL

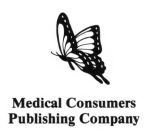

**Medical Consumers
Publishing Company**

Every effort has been made to conceal the true identities of the people and places described in this book, with the exception of myself and my family, and our activities.

Published by Medical Consumers Publishing Company

Those interested in contacting the author may do so by writing to Medical Consumers Publishing Company, 2515 Santa Clara Avenue, #103, Alameda, California 94501

Edited by Kim Peterson
Typography by QuadraType
Cover Design by Kathleen Vande Kieft
Back cover photo by Jay Sousa
Manufactured in the United States of America

9 8 7 6 5 4 3 2

Library of Congress Ctagloging-in-Publication Data
Carroll, Paula, 1933-
    Life wish.
    Bibliography: p.
    1. Carroll, Paula, 1933-   —Health.   2. Breast—
Cancer—Patients—United States—Biography.   3. Thyroid
gland—Cancer—Patients—United States—Biography.
4. Physicians—Malpractice.   5. Surgical errors.
6. Iatrogenic diseases.   I. Title.   [DNLM: 1. Malpractice
—personal narratives.   W 44 C319L]
RC280.B8C387   1986   362.1   85-63449
ISBN 0-936401-00-1
ISBN 0-936401-01-X (pbk.)

To my husband
Steve

Acknowledgments

I am greatly indebted to:

— my husband and my mother who stood beside me and gave me their love and support,

— my many friends and supporters—too numerous to be named individually—who believed in me and helped me to help others.

There is but one rule of conduct
for a man [or woman] . . . to do the right thing.
The cost may be dear
in money, in friends, in influence, in labor,
in a prolonged and painful sacrifice:
but the cost not to do right is far more dear:
you pay in the integrity of your manhood [or womanhood],
in honor, in truth, in character.
You forfeit your soul's content,
and for a timely gain
you barter the infinities.

—Archer G. Jones

Preface

*T*his book is a factual, documented account of my encounter with cancer and the course of my treatment. I have decided to relate my story in order to examine the seeming inability of some members of the medical profession to admit to their failures or to the errors committed by themselves or their colleagues. The repeated mistakes made by various doctors in the treatment of my illness nearly caused me to lose my life and resulted in years of torment, both mental and physical. The fact that I am alive today is not a testament to their compassion or their skill in medical practices, but to my own perseverance and determination.

During the long period of my cancer treatments, the persons named in this book consistently refused to admit to grave errors, unethical conduct, or to the actual illegalities they committed in their handling of my illness. In the interest of objectivity, all proper names, except those of myself and my husband have been changed.

My primary motive in telling this story is not to seek revenge but to alert other unsuspecting patients to the dangers they may encounter in the course of a serious illness. This book is not to be considered an indictment of the medical profession, although it focuses clear attention on the indefensible and unpardonable negligence of certain members of the medical community. Over the past eight years I have learned that the mistakes and subsequent coverup outlined here are not confined to the persons I mention but are found in other localities as well.

I also hope to awaken the sensibilities of those whose professed vow is to safeguard human life through medical treatment. Perhaps I may influence them to accept their full responsibility to protect the dignity and sanctity of each life entrusted to their care. I consider myself to be one of the lucky ones—I have survived to warn others of the pitfalls and to assure them that there is always hope, and help is available. All medical records involved in my case are available to any qualified person who wishes to study the documented facts.

After all, there is more to me than any surgeon can remove. . . .

—Paula Carroll

Chapter One

For over four years, during bi-annual visits, my physician, Dr. Henry Lawton, would palpate a lump in my breast and say, "Everything looks fine, Paula. You have nothing to worry about." Those comforting words produced enough false security to keep me feeling safe until my next six-month checkup. Why should I question his diagnosis? Dr. Lawton was the expert and I trusted him.

Then, in August of 1977, I noticed there was a dimpling condition developing around the lump in my breast. I knew enough by then to know this was one of the danger signals of cancer.

I had never before been troubled by any serious illness, and I had never been exposed to hospitals or surgeons or diagnoses. Indeed, my husband Steve and I didn't even have a "family doctor," simply because we were both in good health and had never felt the need for one. As a child, I had had yearly checkups by a doctor with the local health care clinic. But at the time I noticed this latest complication in my condition, the only doctor I had been seeing regularly was Dr. Lawton, once every six months.

I made an appointment to see him. He examined me, his manner mild and unruffled as always.

"Hmm, how long have you had that?" he asked.

"A week or two," I said. "Why? Is it serious?"

I must have sounded alarmed, because he quickly said, "No, not really. There's nothing to worry about. We'll do a needle biopsy."

Lawton did a needle biopsy, and sent the specimen to an out-of-town lab that took ten days to return the results.

When he finally phoned me with the results, he said, "Paula, there is evidence of irregular cells. That does indicate a problem."

1

After all these years, he was finally admitting I might have a "problem." Of course, I had no idea what he meant by "irregular cells."

"Do you have a surgeon here in town?" Lawton now asked me.

"No," I said, "I don't have a doctor in town. Why? Do you feel I may need surgery?"

"It's a possibility," he said. Inwardly, I quaked at the very mention of surgery, though outwardly I remained calm and composed. At this point I still believed I was in the "right hands." The alternatives would have been much too horrifying and outlandish to consider. Dr. Lawton now recommended a local doctor—Jeffrey Forbes. In retrospect I should have insisted on a surgical biopsy in 1973, or at least sought out a second opinion after my first visit to Lawton.

That night I went out with two women friends to a farewell dinner for one of them. In the car on the way to the restaurant, my friend Marion, who knew I had gone to see Dr. Lawton, wanted to know how things had turned out. "It looks like I'll need surgery," I told her.

"Oh no," she sympathized. She then asked, "Who's going to do it?"

"Lawton recommended Dr. Forbes."

"No, don't call Forbes, Paula. Why don't you call Dr. Kearny? He removed some moles for me a month or so ago, and I know you'll like him, Paula. He's such a fine person, the kind of man you just know you can trust and depend on."

The name "Kearny" struck a familiar chord at once. I had known the Kearnys for some time and was quite friendly with Norma, the doctor's wife. Because I knew both Kearny and his wife, it made me feel more secure and "comfortable" about dealing with him as a doctor.

I now realize that to know a man personally or socially doesn't necessarily mean he will be the best person in a medical crisis. In fact, it's probably much more beneficial to go to a "brilliant stranger," instead of trusting a less-than-competent friend, no matter how familiar you've been with that person in a social situation. At that time, however, I guess I hoped all my problems could be contained in my home environment. That's where I obtained all my other needs, so why couldn't I be treated for cancer right in my own backyard as well?

Although I didn't let on to anyone else, not even Steve, I was definitely worried after that call from Lawton: the irregular cells, the dimpling; it was all adding up, though I still didn't want to consider the worst possibility.

I also felt, quite mistakenly, that because our town was a small town, these doctors *had* to be good, because mistakes and incompetency that might go unnoticed in a big city could never be concealed here. Actually,

2

the reverse was true. I had no idea how much the local doctors were getting away with, but because of their close-knit "brotherhood," every inequity was veiled in mutual secrecy. In other words, such coverups and agreed-upon conspiracies were much easier to uphold when so many of the doctors knew each other socially.

Later, when I observed how other local citizens related to their doctors, it occurred to me that these men are often treated like gods. They are the pillars of the community. Because of their undeniable affluence and status, these men are the *crème de la crème* of the town. Hence, the deep respect the natives feel for their doctors is nothing short of hero-worship. The many ethnic groups in town are even easier prey for the doctors, who take advantage of their widespread ignorance and naiveté.

And frequently patients find it impossible to make their needs known to the doctor. They may have a lot of questions to ask, but will forget them as soon as they are in the presence of the doctor. This could be due to their own weakened condition or the intimidating manner of the man—or both.

When my friend suggested Dr. Kearny, he was at once so familiar to me that I quickly agreed to call him instead of Dr. Forbes. Now, of course, I can't help thinking how differently things would have gone for me if I had contacted Forbes first.

I phoned Kearny's office the next day and made an appointment to see him later that week. When I saw him, I was newly reminded of how very impressive this man was. He had such presence, he fairly exuded an aura of trust and confidence.

In any case, I would eventually learn, much to my sorrow, that the imperious Dr. Kearny was all bedside manner and no expertise. But naturally I didn't know all that until it was too late. During that first consultation, Kearny displayed such a loving, caring concern for me and seemed so gentle and kindly, his mere presence made me feel calm and "rescued." And as a patient I certainly wanted to believe he was everything he seemed. How could he not be? Even his speaking voice was deep and resounding and full of conviction. However, why I chose to equate all that charm with surgical skill, I don't know. I doubt that much charisma is needed when a surgeon picks up a scalpel. And yet for a long time, I felt Dr. Jud Kearny could do no wrong, even when almost everything he was doing for me *was* wrong.

After he examined me, Kearny agreed to the immediate need for a biopsy. I assumed this would be a fairly simple procedure, and as Kearny didn't say anything to make me think otherwise, I asked him to schedule the operation on a Thursday. That way I could return to work in Steve's office on the following Monday, as I had to train a new office assistant. Kearny smiled and said, "Thursday will be fine." That's when he first mentioned—in a very offhand manner—that he'd be doing a one-step procedure. Although he did describe exactly what he meant by that, he wasn't very emphatic about it and at the time I didn't let it sink in. "I'll do the biopsy," he said, and then, as if it were a mere after-thought, he added, "If I find a malignancy, I'll perform the mastectomy immediately afterwards."

But I didn't want to dwell on the word "malignancy." I was certain they would find nothing wrong, and I'd be off the table and out of the hospital in record time.

I now know I should have asked more questions. And even when I didn't, Kearny should have volunteered much more information. He should have impressed on my mind the very real possibility of a malignancy, so I would know exactly what might happen to me on the operating table. He should also have told me that I really had a choice, that I didn't have to agree to his one-step procedure. I could let him do just the biopsy, then wait and learn the results, thus allowing time to prepare myself and my family for the ultimate mastectomy.

Instead, Kearny gave me the impression this was a compulsory procedure, or that this was how it was always done and that I had no alternative. In short, it was a case of a doctor taking advantage of the naiveté of a patient. Actually, very few women are experienced in this sort of situation. For us, it is usually a "first time" ordeal. Hence, we have no past precedents to compare it with. But doctors have been through the same situation many times in the past; thus, it is their duty to educate their patients thoroughly before they take scalpel in hand.

Ironically, though I didn't know this until much later, even if I had asked Kearny to wait, telling him I wanted a second opinion, I wouldn't have been able to get one at that time. The fact that I had already chosen him as my surgeon locked me into the relationship. This is the way it works in our medical community: it is an unwritten law that once you commit yourself to a doctor in town, no other doctor will touch you, regardless of your wishes in the matter. I would have had to go out of town for a second opinion.

I had to sign certain documents—release papers—wherein the term "modified radical mastectomy" was clearly mentioned. The documents stated this procedure would be performed if a malignancy was found. However, I was too full of indomitable hope and faith to read the fine print in those papers, or really consider the possibility that I might actually need that mastectomy. I guess I hoped that if I didn't admit this pos-

4

sibility to myself, it could never become a reality. I now know that such blind reasoning has no place when you're about to be wheeled into surgery. In other words, wishing will not make it so, not when a cancerous malignancy is involved. Even though I kept myself under control so that Steve wouldn't worry, underneath that brave facade I was terribly frightened. And yet, despite my inner dread, I kept reminding myself that the latest cancer statistics were in my favor. I had read that seven percent of all breast lumps were malignant. To me, that meant I had a ninety-three percent chance to survive this surgery without the need of a mastectomy. How I held on to that thought!

Meanwhile, when I was admitted to the hospital on the designated day, Steve was quite aware of what might happen to me in Kearny's operating room. He knew exactly what "one-step procedure" implied. But we didn't talk about it. As he would do from now on, Steve would take all his cues and signals from me, waiting for me to talk about it first. And since I knew it would only worry him more if I discussed it, neither of us voiced our fears.

When I knew Steve had a previous business appointment on the day he took me to the hospital—he had to drive out of town for a conference—I insisted that he keep that appointment and "just drop me off at the hospital on the way, I'll be fine." Actually, whenever I have something serious to accomplish that involves me alone, I prefer to do it without any help or witnesses. I find I can handle my own predicaments much more easily than I can handle other people's fears about me. On my own, dealing with problems becomes much less of a burden for me. I don't have to spread the anxiety around; instead, I keep it contained within myself.

By now I had already learned that the most unpleasant experiences in life are those one must face alone. In the final analysis, you are the one who must deal with this personal crisis, whatever it is, since it is happening to you, not to anybody else. Others can sympathize and show that they care, but there's a limit to how much of the pain your loved ones can really share with you. In the end, you fight a very private battle.

The hospital left much to be desired when it came to service and organization. I was scheduled to go into surgery at eleven o'clock in the morning, so I had been admitted to the hospital the day before. Before surgery, of course, I was given no food or water. The woman sharing the room with me had fallen and broken her arm and on the day of my surgery she was waiting for her sons to pick her up. She was unable to dress herself because of the cast, so I got up and helped her dress. She had been ringing for a nurse for the longest time, but no one responded. She was released at about eleven that morning. I was scheduled for surgery at that hour, but I was completely forgotten until two in the afternoon. Finally, a nurse came in, brusque and businesslike, and gave me my pre-op shots and took me in for surgery.

The next thing I remember, I was coming out of the anesthetic, and I could see a curtain draped all around me, and it wasn't at all familiar to me. Then I saw Steve standing at the foot of the bed, his face streaked with tears. To see my strong, brave husband weeping told me everything I needed to know.

"How long was I in surgery?" I asked him.

"Almost four hours," he said.

Then I had no doubt as to what had happened, for I knew a mere biopsy would not have taken that long. I told myself I would not have to worry anymore, for the worst had already happened and I was still alive.

I started to cry. Then I dozed off. . . .

Chapter Two

ven after my surgery, I failed to identify Dr. Lawton's years of negligence and mishandling as the reason for this operation. I was later told that Lawton had assisted Kearny with my operation, though I never saw him, either before or after. Because he never came to see me, I felt there must have been some conflict between him and Dr. Kearny. Later, when I finally did see Lawton, I got the feeling there was a definite strain between these two doctors. A couple of years later I would learn the truth from another physician who had, on many occasions, "witnessed" Kearny's cancer surgery technique. This doctor related how Kearny would routinely cut into cancerous tumors during surgical biopsies. Kearny always replied to this doctor's protests with a casual "Don't worry—everything'll be alright."

"Unfortunately," said the doctor, "more often than not, everything wasn't alright for the patients. When the surgical field was flooded with cancer cells, Kearny's negligence caused an operable, curable cancer to become widespread and metastatic."

According to this doctor's eyewitness account, many persons needlessly died because of Kearny's failure to follow the basic standard of cancer surgery. This standard dictates that *all* of the cancerous tumor be removed, *along* with adequate healthy tissue surrounding the tumor to avoid the seeding of cancer cells.

Had Kearny attempted to use this inept procedure on me? Did Dr. Lawton protest to Kearny? This may have caused the obvious strain that existed between these two doctors.

Understandably, after treating me ineptly for over four years, Lawton must have felt it was just too abrupt and brutal to do what Kearny did to me in only four hours. It was, of course, customary for the referring doctor to assist with the operation, for which Lawton was paid a fee of 175 dollars. As for Kearny's fee of 850 dollars, it wasn't until the next morning that I learned how he meant to use it: to finance a vacation. I should have been told in advance that he would be unavailable immediately after surgery; I would have appreciated the opportunity to talk over the operation and my future prognosis with him.

But at seven o'clock on the morning after my surgery, Dr. Kearny stood at my bedside, smiling. He had come to bid me goodbye. I remember thinking how very nice he looked, for he dressed so elegantly, always in the height of fashion.

"Paula," he said, his tone as low and soothing as ever. "If I had known how this was going to turn out, I would have cancelled my trip. . . ."

I looked up at him. "What trip?"

"Now don't you worry about that, brave lady," he said. "I'll only be gone for awhile."

When he said that, I assumed he would only be gone for the weekend. As it was Friday, I thought he'd be back on the following Monday. Little did I suspect that he would be out of town for more than ten days.

"I'll keep you in my prayers, Paula," he was saying. "But I'm sure you'll be perfectly alright. And one thing's for sure: you really have a husband who loves you."

Of course, I was still very groggy, so I just murmured, "Yes, I know Steve loves me. . . ."

"My colleague, Dr. Butler, will take over for me while I'm gone," he said. He continued to praise my loving husband, my caring friends, my luck—in fact, he was hoping to distract me from my immediate dilemma and disguise his eagerness to get out of town so quickly. In his hand he held a little booklet, a gift to me from his wife. "I didn't know you knew Norma," he said. His tone was still so light and bantering, you'd think he and I were idly chatting at a garden party.

"She sent this book to you," he continued, handing it to me. It was entitled *Faith Is*. It was a colorfully illustrated inspirational book, and it, too, succeeded in diverting me from the fact that the man who had just performed a mastectomy on me was now eager to leave on his vacation.

At this time, even if I had known in advance how long Kearny meant to be away, I wouldn't have questioned him, for I was still convinced I was getting the best care, certain that a doctor like Kearny must know what he was doing—after all, he had had such a long and distinguished career. However, when I met Kearny's assistant, Dr. Butler, I was in for a rude awakening.

Dr. Ted Butler was undeniably ill-mannered. The next day, about fifteen hours after surgery, Butler came into my room and casually announced that I might need skin grafts.

No one had even mentioned this possibility to me before, so I asked, "Why wasn't that done at the time of my surgery?"

"Oh well," he shrugged, "sometimes the skin dies and sloughs off and skin grafts are necessary." He said all this without a smile; his manner was brash and abrasive. Butler did not have Kearny's charismatic bedside manner, and I could have used some of the surface charm and subtlety at that moment, no matter how misleading it might have been.

When he first came in to my room, he did not correct my assumption that he had come to change the bandage. In fact, he simply removed it. "You can look at the incision now, if you want to," he said.

"No," I said. "If you don't mind, I'd prefer to wait." If he hadn't been so insensitive, he might have known I wasn't quite ready to view the damage. I'd had more than sixty stitches and the idea of seeing myself at this point was not exactly what I needed to help boost my postoperative morale. Dr. Butler should have known this; I have since learned that most surgeons leave the bandages on for at least three or four days after surgery, primarily for psychological reasons. This delay gives the patient time to adjust to the whole trauma and is a particularly helpful therapeutic device following a mastectomy as it provides a time of transition when the patient can gracefully become accustomed to this new change in her life.

As for Dr. Butler, he simply removed the bandage and left me alone, unbandaged, knowing I would look at myself after he left me. He was really behaving as if this whole episode should be just as routine for me as it was for him. However, as I soon learned, Butler's abrupt treatment also reflected the attitudes of the rest of the hospital staff. Later, after I completed a great deal of personal research on cancer and cancer patients, I learned how callously so many of the nurses and other staff members treat cancer patients.

I have now come to the conclusion that many members of the medical community are terribly afraid of this malady—the Big C—which is why an alarming number of doctors are squeamish about dealing with cancer patients. They may tend to the basic physical needs, but they will not stay in the room and chat or try to befriend the patient. Of course, the medical experts claim it is standard policy to avoid emotional involvement with patients who may be terminal. But I feel differently about this. There should be a happy medium between being abrupt and cruel and offensive, and not getting too chummy. The patient should never get the feeling of being "dismissed," and that's exactly how I felt.

With the exception of one nurse who was unusually thoughtful and attentive, I usually felt abandoned by the nurses. Perhaps being around a mastectomy patient reminded them how easily this might happen to them, and they didn't want to dwell on that possibility. One of the nurses had openly stated to others, "If I ever needed a mastectomy, I'd kill myself first." (Even the wife of one of the staff doctors had refused to have a mastectomy, and as a result she died of cancer.)

After Dr. Butler removed my bandages and left me alone in my room, the inevitable happened: I had just been told I would need skin grafts, and now I saw the fresh wound that used to be a part of my body—only fifteen hours after surgery. If Butler had put on a fresh bandage immediately, I'm sure I would have waited several days before subjecting myself to this shock. Naturally, I was horrified and disturbed by what I saw. The twelve-inch diagonal incision was puffy and red and was held together with dozens of black sutures. At the lower end of the incision a tube had been inserted to drain off the fluid.

Viewing myself, the true significance of my surgery became agonizingly clear: here was the evidence for me to see, in the flesh. I was as shattered by this sight as any woman would be. A part of me was gone forever, and it was totally irrevocable, something I would never be able to change. I felt mutilated and incomplete, and for a time it was impossible for me to reconcile myself to the new reality that would now be "me."

It was in that moment, so soon after surgery, that I was forced to view and to accept my new identity: I was a "cancer patient." That is when I vowed to make something beautiful out of this experience. Inwardly, of course, I knew I really hadn't changed—I knew it with a deep conviction. But in the beginning I also knew it wouldn't be easy for me to transcend that first shock, the stigma of what had happened to me. I knew that eventually I would come to the conclusion that not everything in the world had changed for me, merely that one minor "rearrangement" had occurred.

I knew I would learn to live with that in the same way I had conducted my life before this happened. I'd tell myself: "I have lost a breast—nothing more. Not my mind, not my husband or my home or my work or anything else that made life such a rewarding challenge for me. All the rest, all the wonder, is still "there" for me, still intact. . . .'"

Perhaps it was true that from a doctor's standpoint, I was now and forever a "cancer patient," no matter how the prognosis shifted from year to year. But I still believed I was more than a doctor's diagnosis, a lot more.

Later I would realize how differently other people would relate to me, and how the perceptual image of me would change in the eyes of those who knew what had happened to me. Actually, it didn't matter nearly so much how well *I* adjusted to the surgery, for I would still have to deal with the attitudes of others. In time, this became a greater challenge than facing my personal readjustments. People have various ways of reacting to cancer: they will either give you "special" or pitying treatment, which I didn't want, or they will ignore you completely, as if they don't want to be reminded that this could also happen to them.

Steve came to visit me every morning, bringing me a rose from our garden each day. At my request on that first day after surgery, he also brought me a paperback copy of the book *First You Cry*, which I had noticed on the newsstand, though it would seem I was absorbing this sort of first-hand information a little late.

I wanted to read this book and see how another woman had weathered the same crisis. I remembered seeing the film version of the book on television, and though I was moved by the dramatization, it was difficult for me to identify with that woman. What she was going through seemed so safely removed from my world. Now, however, I could certainly identify with her.

I read a great deal of the book that night. Butler was making his rounds that night and happened to enter my room while I was reading. From his attitude, I saw at once that he did not approve. He reacted as if I was actually reading something subversive.

To my amazement, he got furious with me.

"What are you doing with that ridiculous book?" he shouted. "Who in the world would bring you a book like that? There are a lot of thoughtless people in this world. . . ."

"Yes, I agree," I said quietly. "The thoughtless person was my husband, and he brought it to me because I asked him to, and also because I've got a lot to learn about what's been happening to me. I want to know how other people have handled the same problem I'm facing. I want to be able to relate to someone. Don't you understand?"

"Well, you won't learn anything by reading trash like that," he went on. "That woman's just hysterical, overdramatizing her condition the way all women do!" He paused and stared coldly at me. I felt sure it had just occurred to him that, unlike "all women," I was quite definitely *not* overly dramatic about my condition. "Anyway," he said, "if you have any questions, it would be best to ask an expert, instead of going around reading junk like that." On and on he went, reprimanding me, downgrading the book.

Before he was finished, Dr. Butler did everything but forbid me to read the book. At any minute, I expected him to tear it out of my hands.

Naturally I was devastated by Butler's attitude, not to mention the gall of the man to judge what I chose to read. As it happened, Steve had been visiting me that night, but had stepped out to get a container to water the many plants that had been sent to me by my friends. It was while Steve was out of the room that Butler had come in and denounced me for reading the book.

When Steve returned, to my surprise, Butler treated him with all the tact and diplomacy he should have extended to me as his patient. His whole manner changed from vicious to congenial in an instant. He patted Steve on the back, smiled, and said, "Don't worry, you'll be just fine. You have nothing to worry about. I know a lot of guys who've been through what you're going through." Then he left us alone.

"Nice guy," Steve said, giving me a smile.

"Oh really?" I said softly. Then I told Steve how the doctor had blasted me for reading my book.

Infuriated, Steve swore and made for the door. "Wait till I have a talk with that guy," he said. "Why, I'll . . . I'll throw him out of the window!"

"Steve," I said, "would you please come back here and arrange those plants in the corner? They look terribly crowded over there; they are all so close together. . . ."

He turned and gave me a grin. "Okay, honey, if you're not mad, I'm not mad. But imagine the nerve of that guy, trying to tell you what to read. Why, that is unadulterated censorship."

"Well, actually, all he succeeded in doing is whetting my curiosity even more," I said. "Any book Dr. Butler hates as much as all that must be a prizewinner, so I won't close my eyes tonight until I've finished it."

And sure enough, by the time Butler came to see me the next morning, I had already finished *First You Cry* and had gone on to a book of inspirational poetry by Dr. Robert Schuller.

Butler eyed the volume of poetry and then, taking it out of my hands, said, "Now *that* book I approve of."

Of course, I should have said "Who cares?"

Chapter Three

On the following Monday morning, Dr. Butler came in and told me that my test results had come back from the lab. Naturally, I was eager to learn the outcome, and I'm sure he knew that.

"Sorry, Mrs. Carroll," he said, not sounding in the least sorry, "I can't discuss the results with you."

"But . . . why not?"

"Because I'm not your doctor," he said. "You'll have to wait until Dr. Kearny comes back."

"And when will that be?" I asked.

"Oh, another eight or nine days."

This was the first time I knew how long Kearny planned to be away. I wondered why he hadn't told me that when he so graciously bade me goodbye the morning following my surgery. It didn't seem that he'd been called away on an emergency, for this trip had obviously been planned for some time. He should have referred me to another surgeon, one who would remain with me and be available to give me my follow-up treatment afterwards. I remembered that this was how it had been done when a friend of mine needed a mastectomy. Originally, she had gone to her primary doctor, but knowing he was due to leave town in a few days, he sent her to another surgeon who would be on hand after her surgery. Of course, that friend had not gone to Dr. Kearny. And yet, I had another very dear friend in town, Doris Fredrickson, who'd had a mastectomy about ten years earlier, performed by Kearny and his associate, Dr. Robins. Dr. Robins was Doris's doctor, so he performed the surgery, while Kearny assisted. The fact that ten years later she was still well and thriving had been a source of great encouragement for me, though it would

13

later occur to me that ten years ago, these men might have had a better grasp on their surgical tools.

In any case, Dr. Robins's bedside manner was as crude and tactless as Dr. Butler's, judging by what Doris told me about that experience. When she was coming out of the anesthetic after her mastectomy, Dr. Robins told her bluntly what had happened, and added this final sentiment: "You can live or you can rot. The choice is yours."

I couldn't imagine any doctor being that callous to a patient after such a traumatic operation. It had to be a new low in counseling technique. As it turned out, these unholy three were closely linked together, both professionally and socially, with Kearny supplying all the charm, while Butler and Robins were consistently tactless, blunt, and unfeeling. In time, I would conclude that you could put all three of those men together and still not come up with one capable doctor.

When Dr. Butler told me I would have to wait until Kearny returned before I could learn the results of my tests, I realized I would have to wait a total of twelve days for this vital information. Yet I was sure Butler knew the outcome of those tests. Because this dealt with so crucial an ailment as cancer, I felt it was his responsibility to inform me and also to take whatever procedures he felt Kearny would take—immediately, not ten days later.

Before he left my room that day, Butler gave me this parting comment: "If the armpit nodes are clear it won't mean much because your cancer mass was above the chest and lungs, Mrs. Carroll. If you have a problem, the cancer may have penetrated the chest cavity."

That only confused me more, and I'm sure he knew that. "What does that mean exactly? Will I be given chemotherapy, radiation, or what?"

"I don't know," he said sharply. "If you were my patient, I'd give you radiation."

And he left me with that, knowing that I still had no idea how I would be affected by the outcome of those tests. In similar cases, a patient normally waits about three days for the test results.

Somehow I managed to remain relatively cheerful and optimistic that following week, mostly to keep my visitors from getting depressed. It became a new challenge—to keep my friends and family members from looking mournful when they came to see me. To boost my mother's morale, I even told her of my long-range plans to help other cancer patients as soon as I was well enough. I planned to study hard on this subject, then find a way to help other patients.

Such were my plans, even while lying in the hospital so soon after surgery. I have always had a future game-plan to look forward to, something I could think of as a special incentive. Whenever I'm involved in a major project, I like to know in advance what will be next on my agenda. Knowing there's a new challenge awaiting me offsets any letdown I might have when the current project comes to an end. So now I tried to look beyond those bad days and project myself into a more constructive future, hoping to put this experience to work to help others.

I knew that many women overreact to this kind of trauma, feeling the loss of a breast is far more symbolic or catastrophic than it really is; for some it seems to signify the end of their womanhood. For me, fortunately, a concern for my appearance was never that important. I felt the most precious qualities that made me a woman had nothing to do with my anatomy, for as I would soon learn, the very best of me shone from within. Moreover, in light of all that happened to me, I got to know myself so much better. I discovered for example, that I can handle a lot more than I ever thought I could, and that I'm a lot stronger than I ever realized.

Soon I was able to get out of bed and walk in the halls with Steve when he visited. However, though it's true I have a high pain threshold and don't hurt as intensely as some people do, at this time I was still in a lot of pain and could only brush my hair with my left arm.

By now I had also been taught my physiotherapy, such as it was. Actually, it was so simple, I wasn't too offended that the staff members took so little time to teach me this exercise. It consisted of crawling the wall with my fingers, going gradually higher and higher in order to strengthen the muscles in my right arm. That was the extent of rehabilitative therapy or counseling offered by the hospital.

I was released from the hospital eight days after my surgery, though I still had not been told the results of my tests. However, Dr. Butler had told me that the pathologist's report had revealed that the lymph nodes were clear. Although he didn't explain this more explicitly, the simple word "clear" was enough to make me hopeful and optimistic. I reassured myself that when Dr. Kearny returned he would surely take me under his wing and give me all the post-operative treatment and care I might need.

As you can see, medically speaking, I still believed in Santa Claus!

Meanwhile, just "going home" became a festive and meaningful event for Steve and me. He came to get me, accompanied by a friend who brought a station wagon to carry all my flowers and plants home. All those thoughtful gifts and cards reminded me of how many beautiful, loving friends I had.

On that first night home from the hospital, Steve offered to go out and shop for food for our dinner. But I told him I had a better idea. "Let's go out to dinner, Steve. I want to celebrate."

He stared at me, amazed. "Oh come on, honey, you just got out of the hospital, remember?"

Unfortunately, I did remember, which was exactly why I wanted to get all dressed up and go out, not only to forget what had happened to me, but to start proving to myself my life could continue "as before." I guess some people would think me a little strange for wanting to do this, my first night home after radical cancer surgery, but I felt I still had a lot of reasons to rejoice. For one thing, I was still alive, and I had a husband who worshipped me; thus, I had no intention of withdrawing from the mainstream, not even for a little while.

When Steve was convinced I was serious, his spirit of high adventure soon matched mine.

The next morning, nine days after surgery, as scheduled, Steve and I went to Dr. Butler's office, as he was due to remove some of my stitches and give me a post-op examination. This would be my first run-in with Kearny's waspish receptionist, Tess Sumner. I would later conclude that Mrs. Sumner was easily the most disagreeable person I'd ever encountered. She was even less charming and approachable than Dr. Butler and for some weird reason, Sumner took an instant dislike to me. Why, I couldn't decide. Whatever the reason for her resentments, they showed loud and clear from then on. I felt it was a temporary dislike, however, and tried to always be pleasant to her.

She showed us into Butler's reception room that morning and said gruffly, "Wait here."

"How long will it be before my wife can see the doctor?" asked Steve, who was being even more protective of me than usual.

In reply, Sumner just glared at him for a seething second, then said, "You'll have to wait your turn like everybody else!"

Steve and I looked at each other, as if to say, "*What* everybody else? We're the only ones here." Just before I was led into Butler's treatment room, Steve found time to whisper in my ear, "What a doll! Wonder where she parked her broomstick?"

When Dr. Butler came in, he carefully removed every other stitch, and it seemed to me his manner wasn't quite as abrupt as it had been earlier. He appeared quite surprised at how well I looked. I don't know why he was surprised, since I hadn't had plastic surgery.

"How are you able to raise your arm?" he asked.

"Very carefully," I joked with him, and that surprised him, too. So I demonstrated for him. Although my right arm was still very sore, I showed him how high I could raise it.

Two days later, on a Sunday, I found out quite by accident that Dr. Kearny was back in town. Steve and I saw the Kearnys while having dinner at a local restaurant. He, as well as other friends we encountered that night, seemed surprised to see me out and about so soon.

In any case, I learned that Kearny wasn't scheduled to be back in his office until the following Tuesday, which meant I had to wait two more days to have my first post-op appointment with the surgeon who had performed my surgery thirteen days earlier.

After he examined me, he said, "Well, Paula, you're doing just fine."

"I'm glad to hear that," I said. "What happens now?"

He looked surprised. "What have you got in mind?"

"I mean, what sort of treatment or therapy will I be getting? Shouldn't I have scans?"

"No treatment or scans are indicated in your case," he said lightly.

"Really?" I said, quite stunned to hear this. "Are you sure I need no treatment or scans at all?"

"Of course not. I anticipate no complications in your case. You have nothing to worry about."

"But . . . what about the skin grafts that might be necessary?"

With that, he eyed me sharply. "Where did you get that idea?"

"Dr. Butler mentioned it to me."

"He was mistaken. I assure you, if we had needed skin grafts, we would have done them at the time of your surgery."

I was quite bewildered by this response, because now I also remembered something else Butler had said to me: if I had been his patient, he would have recommended radiation therapy, because of the location of my cancer. When I thought of that, it bothered me that Kearny wasn't going to do any follow-up therapy. It also worried me that he wasn't going to do any scans or blood tests. By now I had read many articles on this subject and had spoken to several friends who had also had mastectomies.

According to what I had learned, there were certain tests your doctor is supposed to do after surgery.

I mentioned these diagnostic tests to Dr. Kearny, and he scoffed at the idea. "Nonsense, Paula, I don't know what you've been reading, but each case is different. Believe me, you're doing just fine. Trust me when I tell you you have nothing to worry about."

"And I won't need any further therapy or treatment at all?"

"None whatever," he said, beaming that expansive paternal smile at me. "Isn't that good news?"

Inwardly, the doubts were stirring, so I wanted to answer him by saying "I hope so." But I merely said, "Of course it's good news, Doctor. You've really taken a load off my mind."

But he hadn't. Not really.

After that visit to Kearny's office, I still couldn't accept that he had dismissed me without suggesting any further treatment. I knew I should have felt optimistic, as this obviously meant they'd found no cause for alarm when they studied the results of my tests. I figured this meant they must have been positive that all of the malignancy was removed during surgery. And yet, Kearny had been so vague about my condition, had spoken to me only in soothing platitudes, telling me so little that was specific.

A few days later I read an article discussing a new book on this subject called *Why Me?*, by Rose Kushner. The article prompted me to buy the book, and my belated education began. It was at this point that I realized how little information is available to the patient.

Kushner allowed her regular doctor to perform only a biopsy. When it came to more specialized surgery, she wanted a real cancer expert. She considered the one-step procedure to be "barbarism right out of the Middle Ages."

She further stated that the average surgeon may perform two cancer operations a month and that furthermore, his overall understanding of this disease is very limited, because most of his time is spent treating other, less crucial ailments. She also went into detail as to what you should expect and demand of your doctor following surgery, discussing the follow-up tests and the post-operative treatment you should get—none of which Kearny had offered me.

After reading her book, my first reaction was, "*Now* she tells me!" But after further study and consideration, I decided it needn't be too late for me after all; in time, I became convinced that this book saved my life. Luckily, I still had time to avoid other blunders and discrepancies.

Of course, I knew better than to confront Kearny with Kushner's book, for I was sure he would dismiss it as the ranting of some hysterical or menopausal woman, in much the same way Dr. Butler had attacked *First You Cry*.

Chapter Four

*I*n early November of 1977, only two weeks after my surgery, I went back to work at the office. The woman who had been with us for two years was leaving, so I felt I was needed to train her replacement. Besides, I didn't want to stay home playing invalid any longer. I missed working with Steve, and I was too conditioned to staying active. I also felt strongly motivated to get my life in order again and resume a normal pattern of living.

One evening a few days later, while I was lying at home on the couch, I turned my head and felt a catch in my neck. I fingered the area and at once felt a lump.

I went to see Dr. Kearny on November 14th, and during a routine post-op checkup, I told him about the lump I had noticed.

Kearny examined my neck, and at first said, "I don't feel anything."

"You don't?" I said. "It's right here." I pointed it out.

Unable to palpate it, he quickly proclaimed it to be "only a muscle spasm." That seemed like an odd diagnosis to me. I hadn't felt a spasm, I did feel a lump. How could both these conditions be one and the same?

As I later came to learn, Kearny should have checked out my thyroid gland as a routine follow-up procedure after my breast surgery. In the pre-op physical report, just six weeks earlier, he had stated that my thyroid was "normal," which, in fact, was not the case. And yet, even when I pointed out the lump, he didn't suggest checking out the possibility that I might now have a thyroid malignancy. Thyroid cancer is quite rare; only about one percent of all cancers involve the thyroid gland. But Kearny simply called it a "muscle spasm," and once again dismissed me.

It appeared this man was determined to take the easiest way out, no matter how critical the ailment might prove to be.

However, despite these new developments, at this time I was determined to divert myself from my medical situation by building up a new support system and not withdrawing from the sort of activities in which I normally involved myself. I had plans to counsel other cancer patients. In short, I felt I had to be "other-directed."

Steve and I had always enjoyed driving to Reno a few times a year to take in live entertainment. When I heard that both Liberace and Mitzi Gaynor would be appearing in Reno, I told Steve I planned to drive there with a girl friend, stay overnight, and catch both shows.

Steve was appalled at this suggestion. "Three weeks after surgery? I won't hear of it."

He knew that Liberace and Gaynor were big favorites of mine, and when he realized I would have a chaperone in my friend, Madge Crenshaw, he said he felt a little better about the idea, as long as I promised to phone him after we arrived so he'd know we had arrived safely. Madge and I took a couple of days off, drove the 365 miles to Reno, caught Liberace for the dinner show, and made it to Harrah's just in time to see the vivacious Mitzi at the midnight show. It was all such joyful fun, I forgot to be tired.

For me, that little jaunt symbolized so much. It was like turning a corner, for now I had firmly convinced myself I could continue with my life just as I always had, that I could go on building up new memories of recreation and involvement, despite what had happened to me. It was also a great boost to my confidence to know I could still look as good in my clothes as ever.

When I told the doctor about my trip, he gave me an incredulous look and said, "You're certainly making a surprising recovery. How are you managing to hold up so well?"

"Well, when I start to feel depressed," I said, "I remember when Jesus said to Peter 'Oh ye of little faith.' I know we are born to be survivors, and I know I will never face a greater challenge than I can handle."

Tears welled up in his eyes as he listened to me.

I then asked him if I could be fitted for a prosthesis. He said it was a bit soon, then added: "But if you just went to Reno and saw two shows in one night, I'd have to say you're ready for the next step." He also told me he had never had a mastectomy patient adjust so well and so quickly.

I know now that some mastectomy patients refuse to be fitted with a permanent prosthesis to keep from admitting the truth of what has happened to them. But I found it an enormously strengthening decision to make. It becomes very therapeutic to accept the reality of what has happened to you.

A week later, during the latter part of November, I awoke one morning feeling ill and feverish, certain I must be running a temperature. Dr. Kearny had told me to call him if I experienced a rise in temperature, because I had been given a blood transfusion during surgery. In some cases, if a patient has received contaminated blood during a transfusion, there is the chance of contracting hepatitis; a rising temperature is one of the first symptoms of this condition.

At this time I was also feeling some pain in the lower area of my incision, which was puffy and swollen. When I telephoned Kearny's office, I had my first phone encounter with Tess Sumner. This lady hadn't exactly ingratiated herself with me in person, but on the phone she was even nastier.

I described my symptoms to her.

"Sounds to me like you have the flu," she snapped. "The doctor doesn't want to see you for that. Call your general practitioner."

"But I don't have one."

"Then it's about time you get one," she said, and hung up the phone. I couldn't believe such behavior. I had to believe Dr. Kearny knew how this woman worked. I could not ignore the possibility that he used this woman as a buffer, to keep patients at a distance whenever he was in no mood to be "inconvenienced."

When I told Steve how Sumner had behaved, he was furious. He assured me that he would get an appointment for me and phoned a mutual friend, Loretta Barrington, who happened to be a nurse-receptionist for Dr. Victor Post—also a friend of ours who practiced in a local clinic. When Steve told Loretta what had happened, she got busy and made an appointment for me to see Dr. Post. She was shocked that I had been denied the right to see my surgeon, only five weeks after surgery.

I kept an appointment with Dr. Post the next afternoon. Steve and I had known Post and his wife, Jennifer, socially for many years. Actually, we knew them better than we did the Kearnys. The Posts had been neighbors of ours at one time, they had been to our home, and, in fact, for a long time Steve had been led to believe Victor was a good friend of his. However, until now I hadn't realized he was a surgeon; I had always thought he was an internist. However, I did know that Post's brother, Milton, was one of the hospital administrators, and I had always admired these two for their apparent dedication to medicine. My feelings of admiration were soon to diminish.

The next day when I saw Dr. Post, he agreed that Mrs. Sumner's behavior was outrageous. At his instructions, Loretta stated in his record that I had been refused an appointment to see my surgeon only five weeks after surgery.

Dr. Post checked my temperature and said, "Paula, I really feel you've had the flu. But you're practically over it by now, so it's too late for an antibiotic to help you." When he checked my incision and saw how swollen and red it was, he said, "I think that's just a buildup of fluid." He seemed a bit uneasy, knowing I was Dr. Kearny's patient, as he said, "It's really too bad you didn't get through to see Dr. Kearny. Actually, I shouldn't even be checking your incision, because you are not my patient." Knowing that Kearny had been my "surgeon of record," Post didn't even ask me to take my bra off, but just checked the lower part of the incision, and with definite hesitancy.

This was my first encounter with "the system": a network of supportive secrecy that links these doctors. Post was actually afraid to go over Kearny's handiwork, lest he infringe on another doctor's territory. In fact, at this point that's exactly how I started to feel: more like territory than a human being. But I was stepping into this "world" completely cold, for as yet I had no idea what lay ahead.

"While I'm here, Doctor, would you please check this lump in my neck? When I pointed it out to Dr. Kearny, he said it was a muscle spasm."

Post checked it, then frowned, "How long have you had that?"

"I first noticed it several weeks ago."

He did not comment on this, neither agreeing nor disagreeing with his colleague's diagnosis. Instead he said, "I think you need a scan and a sonogram." Then he had me drink some water, feeling the lump in my neck as I swallowed.

He nodded. "Yes, Paula, you've definitely got something there that must be checked out."

I knew that, of course, but to hear it from a doctor felt a lot better than simply being dismissed. I had the thyroid scan done, and the next day Dr. Post called me on the phone and gave me the news.

"The results revealed a cold thyroid nodule, Paula," he said.

"What does that mean?"

"The possibility of cancer."

He told me this news on the phone. I returned to Post's office later that week and had the sonogram done there, after which he asked me to come in and get the reports, as he was now sending me back to Dr. Kearny "for surgery." It was shock enough that a "cold nodule" could mean cancer. Now Dr. Post was blandly suggesting I might need more surgery, only six weeks after my mastectomy.

Actually, at this point I would have preferred that Dr. Post take over and perform whatever additional surgery I might need. When I saw how reluctant he was to infringe on Kearny's "territory," I was afraid even to suggest it. But I mustered up the courage and asked, "Would you please do the surgery?" I did not yet understand the rigid structure of protocol that linked Post and Kearny.

He answered, "No, Paula, I am going to have to send you back to Kearny."

It disturbed me that I did not have the right of free choice. Their priorities should have been my health and welfare, not a wish to avoid stepping on toes or breaking unwritten rules by treating another doctor's patient. Now that it was inevitable that I return to Dr. Kearny, it meant I'd be subject to Mrs. Sumner's insults once more, whenever I phoned for an appointment. But I found a way to bypass this: knowing that Sumner went out to lunch at noon, I phoned while she was out and dealt with her relief receptionist.

When I finally saw Dr. Kearny, he read Dr. Post's report. Instead of commenting on my symptoms, or even asking how I felt, Kearny's first question was: "Why did you go to Dr. Post?" He was angry. That was clearly his primary concern.

"I tried to see you, Dr. Kearny, but I was refused an appointment."

"Who refused you an appointment?"

"Mrs. Sumner," I said.

"Nobody refuses my post-op patients appointments," he went on, but his tone had drifted off, and somehow I felt he wouldn't even mention it to her. The woman had been working for him so many years, I'm sure her obstreperous disposition wasn't any news to him. He changed the subject fast. "Now tell me, Paula, when did you discover that thyroid nodule?"

That question really stumped me for a moment. I wondered if a surgeon of Kearny's reputation could possibly be absent-minded. I had to remind him. "Don't you remember, Doctor, I pointed that lump out to you during my last visit, and you called it a muscle spasm."

That obviously took him by surprise. He seemed nervous and edgy. Then he insisted that the lump had changed since he had last seen it, though I knew—and I'm sure he knew, as well—that it had not changed. He was simply saving face. The tests Dr. Post had done were conducted only five days after Kearny had last seen the lump, which was proof that it hadn't changed.

Having caught Kearny in this outright lie greatly disturbed me. Whereas before this I had only been doubtful and uncertain about him, now I became downright suspicious for the first time. How could I trust a doctor who would lie about such an important issue? I was upset over his reaction; I had an impulse to pick up all my records and get out of there. But where would I go, if every surgeon in town thought of Kearny officially as my one and only "surgeon of record?"

It disappointed me to see that Kearny was not quite the dedicated humanitarian I had thought him to be. It was becoming quite clear that he was incapable of admitting his mistakes.

"Well, Paula, I wish I didn't have to say this, but it looks like you will have to undergo further surgery. But it's not going to be anything serious. I believe we'll find nothing more than a benign nodule."

I had the feeling he was only willing to perform this surgery because Dr. Post had already diagnosed my condition and had done those tests. As it was now a matter of record, Kearny couldn't very well avoid it. I felt sure that if Post had not recommended surgery, Kearny would not have chosen to perform this operation. He would have just let it go; he was *that* irresponsible. He almost seemed to ridicule the idea that this was anything serious, though the tests had clearly indicated the possibility of cancer.

It was already December 6th when I was given this news, so I asked Kearny if we could postpone the surgery until after the holidays. I was scheduled for surgery on Friday, January 13th. Before I left his office that day, Kearny said he would have Mrs. Sumner schedule the appointment for me at the hospital.

When Sumner called me at home later that afternoon, she announced my surgery date with all the finesse of a top sergeant, then hung up the phone. From her tone, you'd think she had just scheduled me for an execution. Since she was being even nastier than before, I wondered if Kearny hadn't reprimanded her about her rudeness after all.

Chapter Five

*D*uring that holiday season, I could tell that my family and close friends were worried anew about me when they learned of the additional surgery I would need. That meant I had to fight through their fear as well as my own. Fortunately, having to deal with other people's anxieties kept me diverted from my own.

I had faced the crux of that fear, plunging straight into the eye of the hurricane, and I said, "Okay, you're not so big after all." I knew that through the strength of my faith I could conquer the fear of what lay ahead. Thankfully, my deep faith isn't the sort that makes it easy to give up. It served as an inspiration to find my inner strength and make it work for me.

I soon learned that the worst period of the day for me was early in the morning. During the first week or two after my mastectomy, I absently caught a view of myself in the mirror each morning. Then I realized there was no need to look in the mirror until I dressed for the day. It was much less depressing to avoid looking at the visual proof of what had happened each morning. Thus, I learned to ease into each new day's readjustment more smoothly. Later, when I began to counsel other mastectomy patients, I passed this tip on to them.

Steve continued to shower me with gifts during this period between operations, proving again that he's my greatest fan. He had given me a beautiful canary-yellow diamond ring to ease my recuperation from the first operation. Naturally that would give any girl's morale a boost.

Of course, Steve was very apprehensive about my impending surgery, though he still never verbalized these fears to me. Because we love each other so deeply, we each tried to keep the other from worrying. Although he still tried to match whatever mood I was in, I could tell he was desperately worried about my future, as were the other members of my family.

When I was admitted to the hospital again in mid-January of 1978, Steve had a delightful poster decoupaged for me. It was a fruit tray, and on it was the image of a little boy with a handmade sign that said "You're special." He set it up in my hospital room and it became quite a conversation piece. I knew he had gone to a lot of trouble to find that poster and have it sent to me. I felt a warm glow every time I looked at it.

Before I went in for my surgery, Dr. Kearny explained to me that if the nodule was benign, he would excise the nodule only, leaving a part of the right lobe to produce thyroxine.

Kearny performed the thyroid surgery, with Dr. Post assisting. Immediately following the operation I was very ill, due to an adverse reaction to the anesthetic. I had a terribly upset stomach and was vomiting. I had not been so violently ill after my first surgery. This time, the anesthetic had a completely different effect on me.

When I awoke the next morning, I found the ill-natured Dr. Butler standing over me. Oh no, I thought, not him again! Before my operation, Kearny had assured me he would not be leaving town and that he would remain with me after the surgery. When I made that request, I'm sure he gathered that I had not been pleased with his former replacement. Nonetheless, he was here again.

When I regained consciousness after surgery, I was feeling pain in my arm and I could tell it was very swollen. It turned out that the anesthesiologist had missed the vein and inserted the needle into the tissue. The IV fluid was running into the tissue rather than the vein and this had caused the pain and swelling. My arm was nearly double its normal size.

I pointed this out to Dr. Butler when I awoke that morning and found him standing there. So he took the needle out. I still felt very faint and groggy from the medication, so I murmured weakly, "Oh, you took the needle out."

"Of course I took the needle out!" he barked at me. "What did you expect me to do?" I thought, with his bedside manner, he should be a vet, though I pitied the poor horse that got him for treatment.

"I was only commenting," I tried to explain.

Later, Butler instructed the nurse to pack my arm in ice. Although at the time I didn't realize what a serious blunder the anesthesiologist had made, now I am amazed that I ever survived so many serious errors!

They kept my arm packed in ice for two days, during which time I drank a lot of fluids. Ice packs were alternated with heating pads until the swelling finally went down.

Meanwhile, a few hours after my surgery, while I was still heavily sedated, Dr. Kearny appeared in my room to make this happy announcement: "Good news, Paula. No cancer was found so I only did a nodulectomy. Further surgery was not necessary."

"Really?" I said. "You know that already?"

"Yes, it's true," he said. "We took a frozen section and it was benign."

"Oh, I'm so happy!" I said. "I knew it wasn't malignant, I just knew it! How I prayed for this, Dr. Kearny."

After this joyful announcement from Kearny, I was full of new hope. I was up and walking quite soon, watering the plants my visitors had brought me, talking to other patients, entertaining all my visitors.

Then, six days later, while I was still hospitalized, Dr. Kearny came into my room. Previously he had stood on the right side of my bed, so the light from the window would shine on his face and I could see him while he spoke to me. But this morning he obviously didn't want me to see his face. He walked around and stood on the other side of the bed, with the light to his back, which made it difficult for me to see his face. When I heard his latest report, I could see why he would want to remain in the shadows.

First he presented me with a lovely get-well card his wife had sent me. That was the good news.

Then he spoke, completely reversing his former verdict.

Pointing to my neck, he said, "That was a tumor."

Knowing that a tumor can be either benign or malignant, I asked, "Do you mean the tumor was malignant?"

"Yes," he answered.

I stared in his direction, trying in vain to see the expression in his eyes.

He continued, "I'm sorry if we got your hopes up. It seems our findings were . . . uh . . . premature."

Naturally, I wasn't ready for this new shock. I believe I wouldn't have felt quite so shattered by this news if I hadn't first been given false hope. I later realized this was still another stupid blunder on Kearny's part. He should not have been so quick to tell me the tumor was benign. If he had known his business, he would have said nothing until the permanent section testing was done.

Unfortunately, as had happened so often during my hospital encounters with these doctors, it was only in retrospect that I came to realize how many unforgivable errors Kearny had made in treating me.[1]

However, I did remember that prior to the surgery Kearny told me he would only remove the entire lobe if the frozen section revealed any malignancy; otherwise, he would simply do a biopsy and excise the nodule. I recalled that conversation after the surgery when he said he only removed the nodule because no cancer was found.

With that in mind, I asked him, "Doctor, are you quite certain you took ample tissue?"

And while this was clearly a very serious question, he responded with a lot of silly evasions and meaningless jabber, turning on that tired old "charisma" routine again. "Now, Paula, don't you worry about a thing. Believe me, everything's going to be alright. You have so many friends and loved ones who are pulling for you."

I saw very quickly that he did not intend to answer my question. In fact, he was relating to me as if I were a child.

"You must trust me, Paula, have faith in me." he went on. "Everything's going to be fine."

When Kearny left my room I phoned Steve and gave him the news. He was terribly shaken by this latest setback and broke down on the phone. He, too, had become optimistic when Kearny told me the tumor was benign. By this time, however, Steve had also become suspicious about Kearny's methods of treatment, so he phoned the doctor and reminded him of all he should have done for me that had not yet been done.

"Doctor, it's now three months since Paula's mastectomy, and she still hasn't had any bone scans, liver scans, or even any simple blood tests. I have learned such tests are customary after a mastectomy, so it's time you did what should have been done for her months ago."

"Now Steve," chanted Kearny, "you and Paula are two of the nicest people I know, so don't be upset. Believe me, everything necessary will be done in good time."

"I don't want to hear any more evasions like that," Steve said, losing patience. "There have already been too many stupid foul-ups in this case. So what we want now is another pathologist's opinion."

Whereupon, at Steve's insistence, my thyroid specimen was sent to the Mayo Clinic for study.

Of course, at this point Steve didn't realize that Kearny should have done follow-up tests for my thyroid condition immediately after my surgery. Neither did we know that each type of cancer requires separate and independent scans and follow-up procedures. Kearny knew this but never told us. Eventually he did the tests for breast cancer, but he failed to do the follow-up tests which are always done after thyroid cancer surgery—at least by competent surgeons.

Once, when Steve and I were chatting with one of the nurses, Steve confided in her about the cancer that was found during my thyroid surgery. Unfortunately, Dr. Post happened to be standing nearby, and when he overheard what Steve had said, he whirled about and gave me a sharp look of surprise.

The expression on Post's face convinced me Kearny had not told him they had found cancer. I thought that was odd—after all, Post *had* assisted with the operation. Kearny was obliged to ask Post to assist, as a professional courtesy, because it was Post's diagnosis that revealed the need for more surgery.

Post seemed embarrassed when he realized I had been watching him. So he smiled and walked over to me, pretending to comment on the "clever and original" poster Steve had gotten for me, which I was holding in my lap at the moment. But I could not forget his double-take and felt certain this was the first time he knew about it. Dr. Post also knew I should have been sent right back into the operating room for the proper follow-up surgery, which Kearny had also failed to do.

In retrospect, I think this was when Post began to needle Dr. Kearny for the many blunders Kearny had made in handling my case. It was also at this point that I believe the coverup began in earnest. The local medical establishment was reaching out to protect its own. Dr. Post knew what his old friend Dr. Kearny had done—and had failed to do—but because of their fraternal "code," he had to keep quiet about it. It would seem that this is how these doctors keep a lid on their own ineptitude.

In time, I also learned about the "Godfather" figure who heads the local doctors. Whenever new doctors set up practice in town, this doctor calls them to his home and gives them a list of regulations to which they must conform if they want to have a successful practice here. If they want to make a good living, they will conform; otherwise, they will be treated like outsiders. The doctor who told us of this ritual admitted he had moved out of the area because he could no longer tolerate the pressure. He now has an excellent practice in a different state.

This, then, was "the system" I was up against. And because it was all so covert (for a long time I didn't even know it existed), I never really knew what I was fighting.

But in time, fighting is exactly what I found myself doing—fighting for my life.

[1] The following books and articles were an invaluable resource to me at this time. From them I learned the *facts* about my illness that enabled me to confront my doctors with their errors.

American Cancer Society, "Biopsy principles," *Cancer: A manual for practitioners*, 6th edition, Boston: American Cancer Society, 1982, p. 18.

American Cancer Society, "Surgical therapy: Excision of the primary cancer and regional lymph nodes," *Cancer: A manual for practitioners,* 6th edition, Boston: American Cancer Society, 1982, p. 45.

Beeson-McDermott, eds., "Thyroid neoplasms," *Textbook of Medicine,* 15th edition, Philadelphia: W.B. Saunders, 1979, pp. 1730-1733.

Conn, ed., "Thyroid gland malignancy," method of Joel B. Freeman, M.D. and Farid Shamji, M.D., *Current Therapy,* Philadelphia: W.B. Saunders, 1979, pp. 473-476.

Gordy-Gray, "Tumors of the thyroid gland," *Attorney's Textbook of Medicine,* San Jose: Bender, 1984, pp. 77.59-77.66.

Ketcham, Alfred S., M.D., "Surgery of Cancer," *Ackerman and del Regato's Cancer,* St. Louis: Mosby, 1979, pp. 63-67.

_____. "Pathology of cancer—pathologist's responsibility," *Ackerman and del Regato's Cancer,* St. Louis: Mosby, 1979, pp. 31-43.

_____. "Thyroid and parathyroid glands/Thyroid gland," *Ackerman and del Regato's Cancer,* St. Louis: Mosby, 1979, pp. 421-424.

Schwartz, "Oncology—therapy, general considerations," *Principles of Surgery,* New York: McGraw-PreTest, 1983, pp. 321-323.

Williams, "Treatment of thyroid carcinoma," *Textbook of Endocrinology,* Philadelphia: W.B. Saunders, 1981, pp. 221-222.

Chapter Six

*A*bout two weeks after my thyroid surgery, Kearny arranged to have my breast cancer follow-up tests done. It was a relief to know that the results of both the bone scan and the liver scan were "normal."

After the thyroid specimen was sent to the Mayo Clinic—at Steve's insistence—the clinic sent their report to Dr. Kearny. But he never showed me the report. He never discussed its contents with me, either. When I asked him about it, he only said that Mayo had confirmed what the lab had found.

However, it's interesting to note here that the pathology lab's tissue report following my surgery mentioned receiving only a "thyroid nodule." While Kearny's operative procedure instructions had said "excision of right thyroid nodule," the operating room nurse stated in her report that the thyroid nodule was all that was removed. And Kearny had told Steve and me the day after surgery that all he removed was the *nodule*. It was, therefore, a fact that I had only had a nodulectomy. Dr. Kearny's entry on the surgical report would, however, disagree with what he had told us. It would say that he had done more extensive surgery.

I was disturbed that performing a nodulectomy, which amounted to nothing more than a biopsy, was not *adequate* surgery for a cancer diagnosis. I was additionally disturbed when Dr. Kearny admitted that the pathologist had made a mistake in the frozen section at the time of my surgery. Given these discrepancies, how many more mistakes had been made?

By January 30th, Steve had phoned Kearny several times, firmly demanding that we be given a second opinion. So when this finally happened, it wasn't Kearny's idea—it was only because Steve had pressured him into it.

A friend of mine who had also had a mastectomy by a local surgeon recently told me: "You know, Paula, if a patient wants a second opinion, the doctor will most likely send them to a specialist as far away as Bay City. The patient is not likely to want to keep making such a long trip for future medical care, as it's so far away. Instead, he is more apt to return to the referring doctor. But if you were to see a doctor in some nearby town for a second opinion, you'd be more likely to return to that doctor instead of coming back to your doctor here. You'd be surprised how often I've seen this happen—often enough to know it's an accepted procedure among the local doctors. They really resent having to send you for a second opinion; they want to make sure you come back to them rather than venture to a neighboring town."

This was now about to happen to me, courtesy of Dr. Kearny.

When Kearny told me he would be sending me up to Bay City Medical Center to see Dr. Peter Grayson, he announced it as if he'd just thought of the idea and it wasn't due to Steve's insistence. Dr. Grayson was a surgeon at the Center, Kearny told me, adding: "You'll be in good hands."

I was now becoming increasingly suspicious of Kearny. I was no longer sure I could have confidence in the doctor he was recommending. At this time, I again asked Kearny that pivotal question, "Doctor, are you certain you took ample tissue during my thyroid surgery? It concerns me that you told me you had only removed the nodule."

"Ah, Paula," he said, giving me one of his benevolent smiles. "Don't worry, God's on our side." He patted me on the shoulder.

This was, of course, another evasion. I was so weary of this treatment that I said, "No, Doctor. God doesn't take sides. I'm on God's side."

He looked offended by that, as if I had wounded him to the quick. I suppose for a man of his standing in the community, he felt I was telling him he was not on the side of the angels, but that *I* was. By now I was beginning to have feelings of overwhelming doubt whenever I spoke to Kearny; I suspected him of lying to me repeatedly.

When I drove to Bay City to see Dr. Grayson, he only spent about six mintues with me, so it was hardly worth the trip. All he did was palpate my neck—nothing more. Kearny didn't even send him the surgical slides for review. I was sent to this doctor with a minimal amount of information from Kearny. Thus, when Dr. Grayson said Dr. Kearny had done the right procedure, I wondered how he could possibly have arrived at that conclusion with so little to go on. (Two years later, when Steve confronted Grayson with the proof of what Kearny actually did for me,

Grayson's only comment was, "Kearny and I are friends.") Moreover, knowing that Grayson was a surgeon, I wondered why I had been sent to him for follow-up. He doesn't do follow-ups or diagnostic work, but only performs surgery.

I felt dissatisfied and extremely uncomfortable with his inadequate treatment, as it really wasn't a follow-up at all. Meanwhile, I had hand-carried a letter from Kearny to Grayson, the contents of which I had not seen, of course, because the envelope had been sealed with an inordinate amount of tape. I had no idea what "message" Kearny was relaying to Grayson. However, I now know Grayson was not sent the copies of my surgical report; instead, Kearny had sent him a cover letter explaining his surgical procedure. I found this very peculiar, and began to wonder now if my January 13th surgery report had even been typed up yet. Why else would Dr. Kearny withhold my surgical reports from a consulting surgeon?

One morning in early February I woke up feeling ill. I was running a temperature and I had severe heart palpitations. I felt that part of my problem might be that I was taking too much thyroid medication. During my last visit, Dr. Kearny had told me to increase my dose, even though I hadn't yet taken the thyroid panel blood tests that would determine the correct dosage. And yet, just before I was released from the hospital, one of the nurses told me I should be sure and have Dr. Kearny do the thyroid panel. He never did.

Worried about the way I was feeling, I put through a call to Dr. Kearny's office. Even though I dreaded having to deal with the officious Mrs. Sumner, I felt I shouldn't wait until her lunch hour to call. This time, after Sumner insulted me on the phone, I decided I had to make a change.

I told her how I was feeling and mentioned that I felt it was due to the medication. "Oh come on now, Mrs. Carroll, that's a minor problem," she snapped. "The doctor wouldn't want to see you for that."

"But he's the one who prescribed this medication," I reminded her. She still refused to make me an appointment and she hung up on me.

I phoned Steve and told him this latest trouble I had in trying to get past Kearny's front desk. He was furious, of course, but later that night he and I decided we didn't know or care what sort of problems Kearny was having with that woman, because, for us, it was time to make a decision. I had been having terribly uncomfortable feelings about Kearny anyway, and I saw no reason why I should continue to tolerate the abusive Mrs. Sumner. Her treatment of me had only added insult to injury, and what I needed was expert attention, not a dose of petty office politics.

Despite my suspicions of Kearny, and the fact that I was beginning to feel intimidated by him, I felt it would be more discreet to simply change doctors. In a small community, you learn not to make waves or engage in attention-getting confrontations. But in a way, I was still being acquiescent: I didn't want to rock the boat. I just wanted to switch oars.

Later during that first week of February, I phoned Dr. Post's office and asked for an appointment. I had no trouble getting through to the doctor. My problems began when Post realized what I wanted of him.

"Dr. Post, please take me on as your patient," I was actually pleading with him. "I can't stand the runaround and the hassle I've been given at Kearny's office. It's like being put through some kind of obstacle course every time I try to see that man. . . ."

But Post went into a panic. "Oh, no, Paula. You're Dr. Kearny's patient. I can't touch you."

"Why not?" I demanded.

"There's such a thing as professional ethics," he said. "Now you think about that Paula, and I'm sure you'll do the right thing." He hung up.

"Professional ethics," I thought, confused and frustrated. Did it really mean that the way doctors treated other doctors was far more important than how they treated their patients? I couldn't understand this; I felt I should certainly have the right to decide what doctor I wanted.

I was finally reaching the point of exasperation: I had been refused appointments with my surgeon only five weeks after my mastectomy, and now the same thing was happening to me all over again. I was being refused appointments with Kearny only three weeks after my thyroid cancer surgery. It began to seem that Kearny just wanted all his surgical patients to disappear, so he wouldn't have to face his mistakes.

Indeed, this would turn out to be my lowest point. If it hadn't been for my devout religious faith and my inner core of resilience, I could have been very close to self-destruction during those weeks. I felt abandoned and betrayed by the only people in town I felt I could rely on—the experts.

Finally, a few days later, Dr. Post relented to a certain extent anyway. It must have bothered him to know I hadn't yet received the thyroid panel blood tests, so he agreed to do these tests for me. When I saw him I also told him of the severe headaches I had been troubled with for some time, adding that those headaches had gone on for several years. After my thyroid surgery, they had become more intense.

"Don't you think it's a problem I should have checked out?" I asked.

He had to agree. "Yes, Paula, let's arrange a brain scan for you."

I felt more relaxed after Dr. Post offered to do at least this much. On

February 21st, he sent me to a hospital in a nearby town, where a brain scan was performed. That was another low ebb for me, not being able to sleep and feeling so insecure about my doctors. After arranging my brain scan, Dr. Post refused to accept me as his patient, insisting that I return to Kearny. In fact, when he made that suggestion, he actually looked frightened. I had to wonder what reprisals would ensue if one doctor was found guilty of taking a patient away from another.

Meanwhile, for months I had been having difficulty sleeping, in conjunction with my severe headaches. When I had complained about this to Kearny, he had prescribed Dalmane for me, which I later learned was a very powerful hypnotic drug. At the time he prescribed it, Dr. Kearny told me it was non-habit-forming, and that I would have no problems with the drug. He would prescribe fifteen at a time and when I took them, of course I was able to sleep. Though I have never liked taking such drugs, I was desperate with insomnia and Kearny had reassured me that they were "harmless." But this was a false assurance, and once again, it was the case of a seasoned expert taking advantage of his patient's inexperience.

However, when I told Post of my insomnia, he also prescribed Dalmane, as many as seventy-two capsules at a time, thirty milligrams in each capsule. His failure to enter this fact in his records was illegal.

I felt it wasn't just coincidence that he prescribed the same drug Kearny had prescribed. It should have alerted me to the fact that these two doctors were already in contact about my case. And, like Kearny, Post also failed to warn me of the possible dangers of taking this drug. Dalmane is a derivative of Valium, a drug I had never intended to use. It has been well documented how addictive such drugs can be. In fact, after prolonged usage, one of the side effects is extreme depression and anxiety. Certainly I didn't need anything like that. But gradually I did begin to feel depressing side effects, although, as yet, I had no idea what was causing them. Because I was sleeping better, I assumed I should start feeling better. Instead, I felt lower and more disconsolate every day.

However, because two doctors had prescribed Dalmane, I continued to take it. Later, after reviewing my records, an investigator from the state's Medical Standards Board made this comment about Dr. Post's overprescribing Dalmane: "They gave you a loaded gun and hoped you would use it."

When Post again insisted I return to Dr. Kearny, I really didn't know what else I could do. At this time, my continuing need for medical attention was desperate; it now seemed I had no choice in the matter. I had to return to Kearny.

Again, I called his office during the noon lunch hour, when Mrs. Sumner was not there. When I saw Kearny again on March 6th, for a routine post-operative check-up, he quickly told me that he knew about the brain scan I'd had. Of course, he didn't discuss anything so trivial as the results of that scan—which were "normal"—he just wanted me to know that I couldn't keep any secrets from him. I was annoyed with Dr. Post for betraying my confidence.

About this same time I was asked to be a hospital volunteer. I welcomed the chance to contribute some comfort to other patients.

One day while I was working on the floor as a volunteer, Dr. Post came by. He gave me a smile and a friendly greeting, "How're you doing, Paula?"

"I'm doing just fine."

"That's good," he said. But he continued to look at me in such a curious way, I felt uncomfortable. I had the feeling he knew something, something I didn't know, and something I should have been told. On another day I saw Post's older brother, the hospital administrator, in the cafeteria. I was at a table with a group of women, and he sat across the room and kept staring at me. I got the same feeling about him: I felt he also knew something about me.

I knew I wasn't getting paranoid. I just had this feeling, and it was eerie, as if I was surrounded by all these "experts," who, if they chose, could do whatever they wanted with me. I began to wonder: exactly at what point had I become the enemy? I was crying out but no one would listen to me. No one would help me.

I felt abandoned and betrayed by both Post and Kearny; I knew they were both lying to me. Steve and I confided in a friend of ours, Dolores Foster, who also works with the local medical profession. When we described the situation to her, she strongly urged Steve to take me out of town to a "good doctor."

"I don't trust any of the doctors here," she said. "They're all a bunch of liars. I've seen these doctors get away with too many things."

She told us that most doctors she'd known are highly trained technicians, but poorly educated in any other field except their own. They know only what they need to know in order to make a good living as doctors. In other words, they have "tunnel-vision." At the time, I remembered thinking, "How much greater they could be, if they could be human beings with a full grasp of humanity and all of its diverse needs and problems."

On March 28th, still in 1978, I called an out-of-town medical society which gave me the name of a diagnostician—Dr. Melvin Henderman.

Henderman gave me a complete physical. I made a point of asking him if we could do this on the quiet, as I wasn't sure I had been given the follow-up I should have had. Now, when I think of involving myself in all that subterfuge, I have to wonder what on earth I was ashamed of. Was it my fault I had to sneak out of town to find an honest doctor? I had fallen victim to the common feeling experienced by all too many patients—*I* felt guilty for questioning "honorable" men.

Anyway, I impressed on Dr. Henderman's mind that this all had to be kept strictly confidential, and he agreed. I told him that because I knew so many people in the area, I didn't want it known I had gone out of town to consult with him.

Henderman did a follow-up on my breast cancer, but not on the thyroid cancer. Even at this time I didn't know these two cancers had to be considered separately. I still believed, and as yet, no doctor had corrected me, that one follow-up covered both cancers. Such was not the case.

After my physical, Dr. Henderman ordered a body scan, and this revealed a new development: an adrenal tumor. When he saw that, he told me he would have to send me back to my doctors after all, because they would have to be told.

"They'll have to give you an angiogram to determine if there really is an adrenal tumor. That's the only way to confirm it. But don't worry, I'll work in conjunction with them. I'll be your internist and diagnostician, and they can direct your follow-up there."

Earlier in our visit I had told Henderman how long I had been taking Dalmane. He was appalled that I had been given so much to take. He said it was dangerous to be taking that drug for such long periods of time, and took me off it at once. Only a day or two after I stopped taking those capsules, I began to feel a considerable improvement in my general well being.

Henderman also said he wanted me to have a number of blood tests taken, and that it would be more convenient if I had them done at my local hospital, as it would necessitate about eight hours of hospitalization as an outpatient. Of course, these tests should have been done long ago; it took going to an out-of-town doctor to find this out.

And now, after his examination, when Henderman sent me back to my doctors, I began to feel as if I were wandering around in a maze. Wherever I went for help, I ended up right back in the hands of Kearny and Post. It almost seemed as if it had been ordained that I must remain under the control of the same doctors whose gross ineptitude had sent me seeking out-of-town help in the first place.

I began to wonder when *I* was going to have some choice in this matter, some control over my own medical destiny. Since it was, after all, my body, wasn't it also my prerogative to choose the very best medical attention I could find for that body? And yet here was a totally detached out-of-town doctor who also felt it would be best if I returned to my home town.

It wasn't until much later that I realized exactly why Kearny and his colleagues preferred treating me themselves. After my thyroid surgery, Kearny in particular viewed me as a "walking advertisement" of his medical blunders and negligence. Naturally, he didn't want me taking those mistakes out of town where other doctors could be witness to them. Since I now carried the evidence of Kearny's mistakes wherever I went, he preferred to keep me and my case safely contained.

So back I went . . . to Kearny and Post.

Chapter Seven

could only hope, as I returned to Kearny and Post, that they wouldn't feel too offended or threatened when they found out I had gone to Dr. Henderman. Henderman would be in touch with them, so there was no way I could conceal this from them. On the other hand, they were surgeons, and Henderman was an internist, so his involvement shouldn't really infringe on their territory. I was thinking all this through, trying to find a good way to avoid Kearny's wrath at the fact I had sought another opinion behind his back. I also hoped that Kearny's dedication as a doctor would come shining through for me at last; and once again—naively, of course—I hoped the welfare of his patient would get top priority.

I made appointments to see both Post and Kearny. It was much simpler to see Post, so Steve and I saw him first. This was in early April, 1978. I told Dr. Post that I had seen Henderman and repeated Henderman's recommendations, mentioning the angiogram that was needed. Post examined the list of recommended blood tests and said, "He's not going to find anything with these." This made me wonder whether there was another blood test that *would* have revealed something. If this was the case and Post knew of it, why didn't he suggest it now?

Post then gave me a surprising bit of advice.

"Go back to Dr. Henderman, Paula. The expertise in his town is a lot better than ours, and the equipment is superior to what we have here."

I certainly wasn't expecting to hear that from any local doctor; later, I strongly doubted Post would have made that comment in the presence of another doctor. In any case, I had already made an appointment to see Dr. Kearny, and Steve agreed I should keep that appointment before deciding on my next step. At this point Steve was still willing to give Kearny the benefit of the doubt, which meant that he and I were still treating others as we assumed they were treating us—fairly. In that regard, we were both babes in the woods.

I guess, in spite of everything, I still felt a loyalty to my original doctor, even though I was certain by now that this was a one-sided relationship. True, I was very suspicious of him, and I knew he had lied to me. Yet I didn't really believe they had deliberately set out to do me wrong. I was certain there was no real malice involved and that whatever had happened to me had been accidental.

I had all the recommended blood tests done at the lab on April 10th, and the next day I kept my appointment with Dr. Kearny.

Dr. Kearny entered the treatment room, beaming and magnanimous, and said, "Hello, beautiful lady." By now, his 'paternal aura' had lost its power to console me. I only felt uncomfortable, knowing how much deceit lay behind it.

He was quick to come to the point. "Dr. Post phoned me and told me that you have been out of town. Why did you go out of town?" he asked with anger in his voice.

The town crier strikes again, I thought.

The smug smirk on Kearny's face when he said this actually seemed to be saying: "Regardless of what you do, lady, we're going to find out about it."

"Dr. Post told me all about your trip to see Henderman," he added.

"I wanted a second opinion. That's all. I was also getting tired of having to do battle with Mrs. Sumner every time I wanted an appointment with you," I said.

"Nonsense. Mrs. Sumner means well. You just have to know how to handle her. What did Dr. Post say to you?"

"He advised me to go back to Henderman for treatment because his expertise and equipment are far superior to anything you have to offer here."

Kearny gaped at me, infuriated. I saw at once that this was one bit of information which Post had *not* passed on to Kearny. The whole idea that I would be better off with doctors in another city cast aspersions on Kearny. I was hitting him right in the halo, and I could see how it smarted. He almost fell off his pedestal. But after that initial look of fury, Kearny did regain his composure.

He made an entry in his files, then quietly said, "We'll discuss this with Dr. Post."

He meant *they* would discuss this together . . . in private. I didn't see why that was so necessary. After all, Post had made it clear he didn't want me as a patient; this should have ended any further involvement with me or my case. I should have told Kearny, "Dr. Post no longer has anything to do with my case. And that's not the point here—my welfare and prognosis are what matter."

Later I thought how little their talk had to do with *my* medical condition. In fact, when these men discussed me, I doubt they ever once mentioned my cancer or the treatment I had received, or the treatment I would need in the future. What did all that have to do with the threat to their egos and reputations that my case posed? By now, in their eyes, I had ceased to be a "patient" and was merely a pawn in their deceptive game.

When I left Kearny's office that day, it seemed incredible to me that neither he nor Dr. Post wanted me as a patient, even though they both felt threatened because I had gone out of town to another doctor. Dr. Kearny knew I didn't have a general practitioner, and he only did surgery. What did he really expect me to do, especially when I continued to have such trouble getting in to see him? Dr. Kearny told me that "everything was alright" and that he'd see me "next month."

Another visit just to tell me everything was alright? This man's vocabulary didn't extend beyond that one comment. He gave me the impression that he wouldn't even know if everything *wasn't* alright. For me to return to him would be sheer futility. If I did, in fact, need *any* additional tests and follow-up, he had certainly been given more than enough time to do them.

I felt this had already become a conspiracy, though still an underground one. It was as if the local doctors belonged to a mutual protection society whose creed was: "You cover up my mistakes and I'll cover up yours." That seemed to be their choice in such matters: to cover up, not to correct or repair the damage done. To do that meant they would first have to admit they'd been wrong, and that, it appeared, was inconceivable.

When I mentioned these fears to Steve, I could see he still didn't want to believe it was true. Perhaps he even felt I *was* having emotional reactions. He tried to reassure me.

"No, honey, these men are professionals. There's no way they'd try anything like that. And remember, Dr. Post's my friend. He'd tell us if something like that was happening."

He was even less willing than I to face the unthinkable, if my fears turned out to be true and substantial. Because that result *could* mean my imminent death, it was much too disturbing for Steve to consider.

Now, of course, I had no alternative, so I went back to see Dr. Henderman. After all, Dr. Post had told me I'd be better off being treated by

Henderman, so I was merely taking his advice. I told Henderman I wanted him to do all the follow-ups, including the angiogram.

Henderman scheduled my angiogram at the hospital with which he was affiliated, but then told me he would need my complete records.

When I returned, I immediately signed a release for my records. Steve took the release to Kearny's office, and, predictably, locked horns with Mrs. Sumner. He gave her the release, but she refused to give him my records.

"You can't refuse us those records. According to a Supreme Court ruling, those medical records belong to the patient," Steve said.

To this, she replied, "You'll have to come back later. Dr. Kearny is out right now, and he'll have to okay their release."

Steve left and returned in a few hours. Sumner had the records ready for him, sealed in an envelope with a lot of tape. Steve brought them home, and after I looked through them I realized that three letters were missing. These missing letters could not have been due to an oversight of Mrs. Sumner's because she told Steve that Dr. Kearny had assembled the records himself. The missing letters included the letter that Kearny had sent with me to Dr. Grayson in Bay City, the letter that Grayson sent back with me to Kearny, and the Mayo Clinic letter which confirmed the pathologist's report that thyroid cancer had been found.

I knew those letters had been in my records, because at one point, Kearny had started to read them to me, but suddenly stopped and said, "Oh well, they're saying essentially the same thing the lab is saying."

It disturbed me to find those letters missing. But I couldn't see myself confronting Mrs. Sumner with this accusation. She would no doubt tell me I was having delusions, or that I was imagining things. She would certainly insist that no such letters had ever existed.

Steve and I discussed it, and considered having the records subpoenaed, but at this point it seemed too drastic. Though it was true I no longer trusted Kearny, I told myself there wasn't anything that important in those missing letters, so I let it pass. I thought Kearny might be an uncaring doctor, but I didn't think he would deliberately withhold important, vital information. Before I took the records to Henderman, I photocopied all of them. I did not tell him they were incomplete.

Finally I had the angiogram done at Henderman's hospital. Happily, this test ruled out the possibility of an adrenal tumor. It was while I was there, in the cancer ward, that I met Sister Marion. She got me involved in the Hospice Movement, which is dedicated to helping and counseling cancer patients. When she discussed this group with me, I told her I wanted to be trained as a Hospice volunteer. She promised to contact me when they began the next session of training classes. This was in late April of 1978, and about two months later, Sister Marion phoned and told me they were about to start the classes. This was my chance to make a contribution and help others who were in my situation.

It turned out I was the only trained volunteer who was also a cancer patient herself. As I completed the training classes, I found I was learning a great deal about myself in my effort to help other patients. I learned the meaning of many of the fears, symptoms, and emotional reactions I'd had. And as I tried to let these people know they were not alone, I also convinced myself of the very same thing: I was not as alone and isolated with this disease as I had thought.

I remained quite active socially all during that summer. I was installed as President of my sorority, and Steve and I continued to do a lot of entertaining. Indeed, none of my favorite activities stopped during that period. Steve bought me a sewing machine and I continued to make all my own clothes.

Yet, underneath all this activity, I still held a lingering suspicion that I had been deceived by Kearny and others who had handled my case. Now, at this late date, I discovered that friends of mine who were mastectomy patients all had doctors who were thorough professionals, giving them the maximum of care and treatment. When I compared their feedback to the callous treatment I had been given, I realized more emphatically how I had been cheated. How I envied those friends.

Actually, from the beginning I had regretted not going to Dr. Forbes, the man to whom I was first referred. The majority of my friends in town who'd had mastectomies had gone to him, and now I wished that somehow I could turn the clock back. Of course, as yet, none of those friends knew of the hassle I'd had with Kearny. In Forbes's method of treatment, he was careful to perform all the necessary follow-ups for his patients. As a result, they never had to double-check him the way I had had to do with Kearny. Moreover, I learned that Forbes had been forthright and honest with his mastectomy patients. If only I hadn't gotten sidetracked when I was first referred to him. I could just imagine how differently everything would have gone for me.

One day during that summer, I happened to run across a friend of mine at a shopping mall, a friend who hadn't been in touch with me for some time. She gave me one quick look of astonishment, and started to cry.

"Why Elsa," I said, "what's the matter?" My first thought was that she'd had some sort of an attack, or else she was in some sort of trouble.

"Oh, Paula," she sobbed, "you look so good. And here I thought you were about to die. I've been watching the obituaries every day in the paper." It occurred to me that a simple call would have saved her that ghoulish preoccupation.

I assured her I was doing fine. Of course, I was scheduled for another session on the operating table at this time, though my friends kept telling me I never looked as ill as I was supposed to be.

During my earlier examination with Dr. Henderman, he had detected an enormous uterine tumor. It was to be removed as soon as I was well enough. This, of course, meant I would need a hysterectomy as soon as possible, as Henderman advised me this condition was literally dragging me down.

I thought, "That's all I need—more surgery." Finally, after I obtained three confirming opinions, the operation was performed. This latest surgery was not performed by "an old friend," but by a specialist by the name of Dr. Morrow. This was unfortunate, because, as I later learned, in 1976 Morrow had performed a hysterectomy on a friend of mine. Afterwards, Morrow and his pathologist told her and her husband that she might need additional surgery. According to Morrow, when Dr. Kearny had performed thyroid surgery on her in 1973, cancer was found. They seemed quite certain this was the first time she had ever been told about this. One wonders how they could have been so sure that Kearny had withheld such vital information from her at the time he discovered it.

In any case, my friend was hospitalized the next day and scans and extensive testing were performed. She was then told that Kearny had only done a biopsy on her and part of the lobe still remained. Fortunately, no residual cancer was found in the scans. She now goes in every year for follow-up tests. However, even though she has not gone back to Kearny for years, her general practitioner has never changed her thyroid medication prescription. She still gets it under Kearny's name, as her general practitioner doesn't want his name on it in the event of a problem. When she confronted Kearny about this and asked him why he had treated her so negligently, he became very pontifical. His only defense was, "I'm a good Christian, I'm a good Christian."

When I learned all this later, I had to wonder why Morrow didn't give me his findings regarding Kearny's foul-up of my case only seven months earlier; he certainly must have suspected Kearny's blunder in my surgery. I recently found out that Morrow was severely punished by his peers for having told my friend about this.

Naturally, the thought of facing more major surgery was another shock for both Steve and me. It all seemed to be coming in such swift succession, after a whole lifetime of never having to see the inside of a hospital.

At least, not as a patient. However, I knew this was a vital and urgently needed operation, and I was certain I would feel much better afterwards. I wanted to get it over with so I could forget it and recuperate in record time—which is exactly what happened. I was up and back to work within a very short time after leaving the hospital.

Chapter Eight

Toward the end of October, 1978, Dr. Henderman discovered several lumps in my neck. After further examination, both he and a colleague agreed I should have these nodules biopsied. "Paula, if you had a problem that developed from the thyroid or breast malignancies, this is where the problem would show up," Henderman told me. He urged me to have the biopsy performed at my local hospital, adding that it was best to be at home, near friends and family, during surgery.

I told Henderman I'd find a different surgeon and mentioned Dr. Forbes, admitting that I wished I had gone to him at the onset of this mess. Henderman suggested I contact Forbes when I got home, assuring me that he would confirm the diagnosis, if Forbes wanted to contact him.

Now I was about to face a brand-new runaround. When I phoned Dr. Forbes's office, his nurse refused to make an appointment for me, simply because I had been Dr. Kearny's patient. I explained to her that I hadn't been Dr. Kearny's patient for over seven months and had no plans to ever return to him. "Why can't I choose the doctor I want?" I asked.

"Well, I'll speak to Dr. Forbes about it and get back to you."

Finally, several hours later, she called back and said Dr. Forbes would see me. However, that only happened because, in the interim, I had called a friend of mine who is also a friend of Forbes's. She had called him and spoken to him about me, telling him some of my background and the history of my case. It was then that Forbes agreed to set up an appointment with me.

My first meeting with Dr. Jeffrey Forbes was on November 1, 1978. He had a friendly, comfortable manner to which I instinctively responded. Because I had heard so many good things about him from

47

friends who had been his mastectomy patients, this time I definitely felt I was making the right choice.

Now, of course, the question was: would Dr. Forbes choose me? This question made me very nervous when I first consulted with Forbes; I was afraid I would get another rejection, as I had with Dr. Post. It was really an embarrassing, humiliating position for me to be in—forced to beg doctors for expert and humane treatment.

After a thorough examination, Dr. Forbes agreed the lumps should be biopsied, repeating Dr. Henderman's diagnosis.

"If you have a problem, that's exactly where it would center," he told me. He also agreed with Henderman that it would be too great a risk not to do the biopsy.

After the examination, I went over to the hospital and signed a release to have my records sent to Dr. Forbes. The clerk assured me they would be sent that very afternoon.

So there I was, headed back to surgery again—the fourth surgery in thirteen months!

Dr. Forbes scheduled this surgery for November 14th, in the outpatient section of the hospital. Though it was done under a general anesthetic, I went in early in the morning and left that same evening.

When I returned to Dr. Forbes three days later for a post-operative examination, he was a changed person. He glared angrily at me and then, in an unexpected burst of temper, he said, "Damn it, Dr. Post told me all about your case, Paula." His face was red and drawn with anger.

I had inadvertently stepped into the middle of a raging feud between Dr. Forbes and a colleague of Dr. Post. My coming onto the scene at this critical time further complicated and strained the relationship between these doctors.

A news story would later describe the feud as "Warring Factions" brought on by overutilization of the facilities at the hospital by Dr. Post's colleague.

I was shocked by this unexplained outburst, though I wasn't too surprised that Post had been in touch with him. It seemed he was second only to Paul Revere in spreading the news. I assumed Dr. Post must have told him his version of the story; certainly not the truth. It was infuriating to come up against this wall of prejudice again. I thought: "Why are these men playing their silly games? Don't they know it's my life that's at stake?"

I had deeply regretted that I had not gone to Forbes in the first place, and now that I had finally changed doctors, this was happening. To say that I was totally devastated would be an understatement. Even though I wanted to cry out in pure anguish I managed to maintain my complete composure.

It was even more frustrating when Forbes refused to be explicit when I asked him what Post had said about me. How could I defend myself without knowing what unfounded accusations Post was spreading about me? It further upset me to think Forbes would be so quick to turn against me; after all, I felt he was rejecting me only on Post's say-so.

After Forbes finished with my post-op examination, and his office nurse took the stitches out, he must have realized how upset I was by his outburst. So he patted me on the shoulder and said, "You're a good patient, Paula. See you in three weeks."

I walked out of his office in a daze, numbed by his insensitivity, wondering if there was actually any doctor who cared about my well being. How I kept from losing my marbles altogether at that point is still a mystery.

I remembered the saying, "No battles, no foes, no victory." Statements of truth such as this and my unswerving faith propelled me on to claim my victory. I knew that if I kept pursuing the truth of what had happened to me the truth would be revealed. Armed with my own strong faith, *I would not give up!*

When I discussed this episode with Steve, he and I both wondered just what Post had told Forbes about me. And so, typically, Steve took the bull by the horns and telephoned Forbes. "What's the problem here, Dr. Forbes? Are you under peer pressure because you took Paula as a patient?"

"That's ridiculous!" Forbes shot back. "Nobody puts any pressure on me."

"Then what did Post tell you that got you so angry about the whole situation?"

"I'd rather not say at this point, Steve. It's . . . it's privileged information. Just remember, no matter what Post told me, I did agree to see Paula again, didn't I?"

When Steve repeated this to me after he hung up, I said, "What does that mean? Did Post try to defame me in some way that Forbes doesn't believe? Is that why he's going to see me anyway?" It was all becoming such a muddle.

What we feared was that Post had branded me an off-limits troublemaker. I now know for a fact that when a patient is mistreated by one doctor, that patient automatically becomes "off-limits" to all the other doctors in town. In short, I was a hot potato and nobody wanted to be

49

caught with me. They must have feared I was so fouled-up medically that nothing they could do would rectify the blunders. The damage was already done, so involvement with me could only turn out badly for them.

Thus the edict had gone out from the offending doctor in the case, Kearny: "Hands off. My career and reputation are at stake."

Kearny was threatening his colleagues, telling them they didn't dare try to investigate or reveal any blunder he had made lest he reveal a few of their own. This was the nature of their gentlemen's agreement.

It wasn't until much later that I learned the gist of Post's conversation to Forbes. Apparently he had repeated that conversation to a nurse who also happened to be a friend of mine. She told me what we had suspected of Post was true. He had told Forbes I was an hysterical, neurotic woman and that he shouldn't believe a thing I said. Because Forbes had seen quite clearly that I was *not* an hysterical woman, he became suspicious of Post and agreed to see me. However, had he known at the time how embroiled he would become in this conspiracy, I'm sure he would have flatly refused to take me on as a patient. By the time he did realize how far-reaching the conspiracy was, he was already in too deep to do anything about it.

Meanwhile, after that initial outburst from Forbes, I told Steve I was reluctant to go back to him. But Steve convinced me Forbes was my one and only hope, if I wanted a doctor I could rely on here in town. So I kept my next appointment with Dr. Forbes in mid-December. I dreaded seeing him again, as I had no idea how he would react this time, but to my surprise, his manner was quite amiable and pleasant. In time I saw this was his normal pattern of behavior: I would never know what sort of mood he would be in, each time I saw him. One time he would be warm and friendly, the next he would be cold and distant. It was just something I learned to live with.

During this visit, he asked me what sort of follow-up I'd had for my thyroid cancer. I was so surprised that he was concerned enough to even ask me that question, I felt that perhaps I had found somebody "in charge" who really cared what happened to me. Of course, I told him that I'd had no follow-up at all.

"Well, then I strongly urge you to go see Dr. Gregory Nicholson at Bay City Medical Center. I know you must be sick of hospitals by now, Paula, but I think it's time you saw a specialist on thyroid disorders, and that's exactly what Dr. Nicholson is. He has authored many textbooks on the subject and is known the world over."

My first thought was that one more local doctor was suggesting that I get a second opinion, as long as it was safely far away. Still, I was impressed by what Forbes told me about this specialist and felt he was leading me in the right direction.

When I agreed to see Nicholson after the holidays, in mid-January of 1979, Forbes made the appointment for me.

At first I was amazed that Forbes had been able to put my whole case together without seeing any of my records, which had been withheld by Kearny and Post. Although Forbes had requested my records from the hospital, at the time I saw him on December 18th, he still hadn't received them.

It took three written requests and two and a half months before the hospital finally released my records. Interestingly, it is customary, though hospitals deny this, that doctors must be notified and give approval before medical records are released to the patients. This is a clear violation of state law, which reads that a patient must be given their medical records upon request.

The paranoia that surfaces within the medical community when a patient wants to secure copies of their medical history is *almost* laughable.

As I've mentioned, Dr. Post's brother Milton is an administrator at the hospital. I feel the hospital deliberately withheld that vital material from the time of my first request, on November 1st, until two and a half months later, on January 12th. By then, Forbes had requested the records also, so I had to wonder who was ordering them to ignore our requests?

Yet, incredibly enough, Dr. Forbes had put my case together without seeing those records. That led me to believe this must have happened to other patients of Dr. Kearny. Otherwise, how would Forbes know just what to do? He knew from experience that Kearny wouldn't cooperate in this kind of situation. As it happened, Dr. Forbes had been associated with Dr. Kearny and his associate, Dr. Robins, when he first moved to the area, many years earlier. Having dealt with Kearny before, Forbes knew of the sloppiness that characterized Kearny's procedures. I also think it was when Forbes realized I hadn't had any follow-up after Kearny's thyroid surgery that he first suspected that Kearny had only done a biopsy. Hence, he referred me to one of the world's foremost authorities on thyroid disorders, Dr. Nicholson.

I drove up to Bay City to see Dr. Nicholson on January 15th with new hope in my heart.

When I saw Dr. Nicholson, I could see at once that he meant business—here I wouldn't be dismissed in only a few minutes as I had been when I saw Dr. Grayson at the Center a year earlier.

After examining me, Dr. Nicholson asked, ''Why didn't you have

51

additional surgery immediately after cancer was discovered following your first thyroid surgery in January of 1978?"

I looked at him and said, "You'll have to ask Dr. Kearny that question."

He nodded and said, "You see, Mrs. Carroll, in your case it's unfortunate that both cancers were found so close to one another, because the breast cancer is bound to take precedence over the thyroid cancer. Also, the fact that the large tumor is so near healthy tissue disturbs me. . . ."

"Does that mean you feel I'll need more surgery?"

He smiled. "Well, you know, it has been a year now. . . ." Then he shrugged, as if to imply that it's been all this time, I shouldn't expect miracles. Then he added: "This is an all-too-common failing among doctors: they tend to become complacent about thyroid cancers and neglect them."

He asked that the slides of the thyroid specimen be sent to him. He also wanted to know what follow-up I'd had on the thyroid surgery. As I had told Forbes earlier, I replied that I had been to see Dr. Grayson at the Center soon after the surgery. "But," I added, "all he did was to palpate my neck. He didn't even check the surgical slides."

"You're talking about Dr. Peter Grayson?" Nicholson asked with a tone of surprise. I said yes, that was the doctor I saw. Nicholson then told me he would make a point of sending Grayson a copy of his report.

Nicholson's questions and his overall attitude convinced me I might, at last, find some of the answers to the questions that had been haunting me for the past year. He phoned the lab and asked them to send my slides so he could review them.

The following day I drove to a pathology lab approximately twenty miles away to sign the release for the slides. The lab is owned and managed by a doctor who, at one time, practiced in our town. Even though he has moved out of town, however, his strong ties to the "old guard" remain intact. A friend of mine, Miriam Powell, works as an assistant at the lab, and she asked me, "Who sent you to see Dr. Nicholson?"

"Dr. Forbes."

"Oh. Well, okay, I'll send the slides right out, this afternoon."

I ran into Miriam in the shopping mall later, where she told me she had made new slides of the specimen and sent them to Nicholson. I thought this was rather unusual, as I knew slides had already been made the previous year, in January of 1978, when they were sent to the Mayo Clinic. That was in my mind, though I didn't mention it to her.

It is a *most* important, fundamental procedure for doctors to view and study surgical slides following cancer surgery. This is necessary so the doctors can determine the cell type and extent of the cancer in order to arrive at the course of treatment that is best for the patient. Also, by viewing these slides the doctor can ascertain whether or not adequate surgery was performed (meaning whether *all* cancer was removed).

I returned to Dr. Nicholson on February 12th, and I could sense by the expression on his face that he had something very serious to tell me. I was right. He told me the slides of my 1978 surgery revealed that incisions had been made into the cancerous tissue and not all of it had been removed. I was stunned. Nicholson and the chief pathologist, Dr. Edward Moss, had reviewed the thyroid slides. Nicholson told me it would be necessary for me to have additional thyroid surgery. He said, "Mrs. Carroll, you're too young not to have this taken care of as soon as possible. You have a long life ahead of you, so we cannot leave this the way it is. The surgery Dr. Kearny performed on you was incomplete cancer surgery."

"The way it is?" "Incomplete?" I sorted those words over in my mind. What was he telling me? And exactly what had Dr. Kearny done to me?

Nicholson added, "If more cancer is found you will have to return to the Center for radioactive iodine ablation treatments and scans."

Although I was terribly shaken by this news, I tried to stay calm, remembering I would have to see Steve later that day, as we had dinner reservations to dine out in Bay City that night.

One morning, two days after returning from my visit to Bay City, I went out for coffee with my good friend, Sara-Jane Mitchelson. I told her I needed more surgery, and for the first time, I told someone other than Steve how Dr. Kearny had fouled me up. Sara-Jane and I had been good friends for over fifteen years, so we were very close. I had often heard her sing praises of Dr. Kearny, saying what a fine, upstanding citizen he was, but she had only known him socially, however, never professionally. I could see how it would be easy to like Kearny, as long as you never ventured into his operating room and, indeed, stayed away from his office entirely. As a friend, he would pose no threat to anyone. It was only in his role as a surgeon that he had become a public menace.

It was very healing to confide in Sara-Jane. This was the first time I broke down and cried in front of anyone. Despite her loyalty to Kearny, Sara-Jane was very moved by my situation, and in no time at all she was weeping and commiserating along with me.

That same afternoon I kept an appointment with Dr. Forbes. During that visit, he asked me what had happened between me and Kearny. I had enough sense to reply, "I'd rather not comment on that, if you don't mind. It's all in the past." But Forbes pressed me, asking if we'd had a personality conflict. I said I didn't know, hoping it would get him off the subject. By then I guess he could feel how tense I was, so he said, "That's okay, you don't have to say anymore." I hoped this pointless inquisition was over, because anything that had nothing to do with my medical condition was pointless, though that seemed to be the sort of irrelevant digression these doctors majored in. In retrospect, I believe that Dr. Forbes was trying to find out just how much I knew about my case.

That was the one and only time I ever referred to the treatment I had gotten from Kearny to Dr. Forbes. I felt he didn't need me as a source of information anyway, as he was plugged into the underground.

"Paula, I'm finally getting your case together," Forbes said during that visit. I waited in vain for Forbes to explain what he meant by this. Instead, he switched languages and started speaking what I now refer to as "Medical Ambiguity."

"It's been a long, tough climb, Paula," he said, "but I feel I've almost made it to the top."

I listened to that infuriating double-talk and wondered what on earth he was trying to tell me. Did he assume that sounding like a mountain-climber would enlighten me as his patient? I have come to believe that some doctors are so afraid that you might quote them or remind them of something definite they might have said that they end up saying very little that makes any sense to their patients. I found it very demeaning to be talked to like that, as if I were a babbling imbecile. The one affliction I hadn't yet contracted was brain damage, though most of these doctors treated me as if I had.

Nonetheless, I didn't dare voice any objections to such treatment, because at this point they had me going through my paces like some kind of trained seal. I was in such a state of benumbed shock over all that had happened to me, and so afraid to offend these giants of the medical community, that I did whatever they told me, responding as though I had been programmed. My biggest fear was that they would all refuse to treat me. In that sense, they had me at their mercy, and I was literally outnumbered by this secret society. As yet, I had nowhere else to go.

During that visit with Dr. Forbes, he also shared the letter he had received from Dr. Nicholson, which stated, "The pathology slides reveal poorly circumscribed margins and evident invasions of the capsule of tumor in several areas and the tumor was not very well encapsulated. It's disturbing with a patient in this age group and additional surgery is strongly indicated."

There was no way Dr. Kearny could not have known this the year before. If Dr. Nicholson and his lab technician discovered a year later that the capsule of the tumor had been surgically invaded, Kearny and the pathology lab doctors must have known this at the time of my surgery, because this was the same specimen they had viewed.

After reading Nicholson's letter, Dr. Forbes looked at me and actually said something that was relevant and made sense: "You know, Paula, if you had been my patient, I would have had you back in that operating room right after the cancer diagnosis. You have to make certain you got it all. You just don't take a chance like that." He made a drawing in his medical records that showed how Kearny had only performed a biopsy.

I couldn't get over my surprise at hearing this, for Forbes was actually criticizing Kearny's sloppy procedures by saying what he would have done instead. That was as close as he ever got to admitting that his colleague had made a mistake.

Before I left Dr. Forbes's office that day, his receptionist scheduled me for my second thyroid surgery on March 6, 1979. This time, I prayed that these "experts" were going to keep doing it until they got it right.

Chapter Nine

By sheer coincidence, at about the same time I was due to have my second thyroid surgery, I heard that Dr. Kearny and his wife were planning to take a trip to Northern Wales to visit relatives. They were certainly picking a fine time to get out of the country, I thought. It was my old friend, Esther Morton, who gave me this bit of news. I told her it was "very interesting," and then went on to tell her of the additional surgery I'd be having, due to Dr. Kearny's blunders.

Esther then said a very strange thing to me. "Well, Paula, you know you're going to have to forgive him."

"Of course I forgive him. That is not the issue. He must be stopped. Everyone who goes into his operating room is in jeopardy. I will never have to answer for what he did to me and to many others. You see, *that* isn't my burden. But when I know something or someone is a menace to the safety of innocent people, it then becomes my responsibility to try to do something to correct the situation."

Although I knew my friend meant well, this wasn't the first time I had heard this rather bizarre reaction from people in town who had heard of my grievances regarding Kearny. It was as if, by some crazy fluke, I was the guilty one in this mess, simply because it had happened to me. The fact is that Dr. Kearny was still thought to be "above reproach" by many in town.

On March 5th, I went to see Dr. Forbes for a pre-op visit. At that time he instructed his receptionist to include a copy of the letter from Dr. Nicholson with the records I was taking to the hospital. That seemed unusual to me. Later, while I was in the hospital, walking to the X-ray room for the pre-op tests, I had the opportunity to thumb through some of my records. I read the entire contents of Nicholson's letter, which further convinced me of the seriousness of my condition. However, I was still wary of asking too many questions, lest the doctors got the idea I was considering an investigation. I felt sure that if they suspected that, they would all decide to stop treating me.

Though it may seem ridiculous, I was afraid to arouse their suspicion of *my* motives because, as of that time, these doctors were my only recourse. I had to keep my silence while trying to solve all these riddles.

That night as I was lying in the hospital, a dear friend came to see me. During our conversation she told me that she had met Kearny on the street recently and that he had seemed to be very troubled and moody.

"When I asked him if anything was wrong, he just gave me a sad smile and said, 'All I ask is that you pray for me.' " Then she added, "But in my heart I can't do that, Paula, now that I know what he has done to you."

This was a friend with a true sense of loyalty.

But as I thought of Dr. Kearny suffering with his conscience, I wondered if maybe there were other patients he had recently mistreated. If so, perhaps he was under some kind of disciplinary action.

As I was being wheeled into the operating room, something Dr. Nicholson had said suddenly popped into my mind. He had said that a secondary thyroid operation posed a much greater risk than the first, because of the scar tissue. Not the most cheering thought at that crucial moment, but at least I felt I knew the worst that could happen to me before the surgery, rather than having to puzzle it all out afterwards.

Dr. Forbes performed the surgery, removing the left lobe and the isthmus, as well as the portion of the right lobe which Kearny had left (although he said in his surgical report he had removed it). On the following morning, Forbes came into my room, apparently in one of his warm and expansive moods. He sat down at the foot of my bed. I was still a little groggy from the anesthetic, and I'm sure my resistance was way down. I decided to be very frank with him, feeling the time had come when I had to trust at least one of the doctors.

"You know, Dr. Forbes, as nightmarish as my illness has been, it's the way my case has been handled that has been much more of a shock for me. I'd like you to promise you'll never abandon me." By saying this, I wanted him to know that until now, I definitely *had* felt abandoned by the others.

Somehow I felt he understood, for he seemed genuinely touched by my request. "Don't worry, Paula," he said. "I'll never abandon you. Why, I love you like a sister."

At the time I really believed he meant it. Clearly, I was so desperate to find someone I could depend on, I felt I had to believe in something, had

58

to find some shred of security I could cling to. Unfortunately, I was forgetting that Forbes was still a local doctor, "one of the boys" in other words, and despite my conviction that he was an honorable man, I should have known where his loyalties would fall once his back was up against the wall.

I had trouble sleeping that night, and awoke several times feeling sick and feverish, having to ring for the nurse. Early the next morning, however, I felt much better, strong enough to take a walk around the hospital. As I did, I noticed the place seemed strangely deserted for that hour of the day. I asked one of the nurses where all the doctors had gone. She told me they were all at an important staff meeting. I couldn't help wondering if that meeting had anything to do with my case. Perhaps Forbes wanted the letter from Nicholson attached to my records so it could be presented in this meeting.

Later that morning, Dr. Forbes came in and asked me a question I felt I should be asking him. "What do you think of the idea of going home, Paula?"

"When?" I asked him.

"Right now."

That surprised me, coming only about forty-five hours after the operation. Moreover, Forbes must have read my chart, so he had to know I had run a temperature during the night. Yet, he still seemed anxious to get me moving and off the scene. That seemed odd to me.

I also recalled an earlier request Forbes had made, though because I had other plans, I couldn't fulfill it. He had asked if I could come in for surgery a day earlier than scheduled. Now I wondered if that was because he had wanted me out before this big staff meeting. Or perhaps he was afraid Dr. Kearny might try to visit me. As you can see, even this soon after surgery, I still felt compelled to play detective.

Evidence later revealed that Forbes had called this special staff meeting to report Kearny for his errors in my case. In time, I also learned that during this meeting the staff doctors supported Kearny, which put Forbes in a bad position. It seemed the staff doctors also thought of Dr. Kearny as a kind of living shrine, a man who could do no wrong. Either that, or Kearny had so much on the lot of them, they didn't dare blow the whistle on him.

It was because the staff meeting had gone against Forbes, and he no doubt feared Kearny might try to attempt a confrontation with me while I was still hospitalized, that he was so eager to send me packing so quickly.

Four days later, I went to Dr. Forbes for a post-op check-up. At that point, the pathology lab had given him a report, telling him no cancer was found in the thyroid specimen, which, of course, was news I found very reassuring. However, Dr. Forbes instructed them to send that report to Mayo Clinic, as he wanted a second opinion. This decision also reassured me.

I was so encouraged when Forbes reported these findings, I asked, "Does that mean I won't have to go back to the Center for iodine ablation treatments?"

His reply was typically vague and angry. Once again he was answering a direct question with a silly evasion. Gritting his teeth, he said, "We're not going to quit in the sixth inning!"

I gave him a curious look, wondering what the state of my health had to do with playing baseball. I could not figure out whether his reply meant that I *did* have to go back to the Bay City Medical Center for treatments, or that I didn't. I had reached the point where I really needed an interpreter to decipher these messages. I was still afraid to corner these doctors or question them more directly, lest they hedge even more, or worse, refuse to treat me.

I remembered that Dr. Nicholson had told me the iodine ablation treatments would be necessary if cancer was found during this surgery. But now Forbes was telling me the pathology lab had found no cancer, so I assumed I wouldn't need those treatments after all.

Later that week many of these questions were still not answered, so I telephoned Dr. Nicholson in Bay City. By now, he had been told that no cancer had been found, though this was before the Mayo Clinic's latest report had come back. Nicholson made an appointment for me to see him in May, to have scans and other tests done.

I had another post-op visit with Dr. Forbes on March 26th. By then he had received the report from the Mayo Clinic and started to read it to me. But halfway through, he suddenly stopped and did a double-take. From the look of surprise and horror on his face, I could tell he hadn't read the report until now.

He looked extremely upset. "I'll be right back," he said, and hurried out of the room. He apparently went out to telephone Dr. Nicholson in Bay City. Of course, at the moment I was totally mystified by his actions.

He returned, looking very agitated.

"Paula, can you go to the Center tomorrow?"

"Yes, of course," I said.

He dashed out of the room again to continue his phone conversation with Nicholson. When he came back he told me it wouldn't be necessary for me to go to Bay City the next day, after all.

Finally, Forbes calmed down enough to read the part of the Mayo Clinic letter that had been such a jolt to him.

Dr. Morgan Baker, a Mayo Clinic pathologist, wrote: ". . . This patient is fortunate. I have found residual papillary carcinoma embedded in scar tissue from the previous excisional biopsy. This residual carcinoma documents the necessity of the additional surgery. . ."

Now all my fears and suspicions that something was wrong were confirmed, fourteen and a half months later, and by a different surgeon. I wondered if finding residual carcinoma explained why Dr. Post wouldn't take me as a patient. Surely he knew that Kearny had cut into the cancerous tumor. Was this why Post had been needling Dr. Forbes? This also had to be the reason why Dr. Kearny refused to answer me when I asked him if he was sure he had taken ample tissue. And it had to be why he was so upset when I went out of town to another doctor. He must have feared another doctor would find out, which was also why he withheld some of my records.

Kearny knew that he had cut into the cancerous tumor, disseminating the cancer cells into the blood stream, but just sat back and let the condition worsen, hoping his blunder would not be revealed. Now, of course, the pathology lab had to amend their original diagnosis, in light of the letter from the Mayo Clinic. They were forced to concur with Mayo.

At this point the whole charade had become a kind of tragicomic travesty of errors. Now that both the Mayo Clinic and the Bay City Medical Center were involved, the pathologists knew they'd have to reconsider their original findings.

This was an increasingly frightening time for me. It was certainly no consolation to discover my condition was due to Kearny's incompetence during surgery, or that none of this need have become so crucial if I had gone to a reputable specialist at the start. Again, how is a patient to know who is reputable?

The phrase "residual cancer" meant it had had time to intensify, to metastasize, during all those months when I was being treated so inadequately, when I was given improper follow-up or none at all.

As if all that news wasn't bleak enough, one of my dogs died during this same period. Undaunted, I went out and got a new poodle. We call her "Natasha," and she's a doll, a real clown, as are my two Yorkshire terriers.

Chapter Ten

O n April 30, 1979, I was taken off my thyroid medication to prepare for the scans and blood tests I would have to undergo at
Bay City Medical Center. This entailed a very difficult transition for me,
as I had to stop taking this medication all at once.

This had many effects on my whole system, all of them painful and uncomfortable. First of all, I gained a lot of weight—about fifteen to twenty
pounds of fluid, all of it bloat. My face was puffy and it was difficult to
put on my shoes or wear my rings. Actually, when you are taken off thyroid medication, it literally means you have no thyroid at all, at least in
my case, and thus no means of producing thyroxine. There was no other
medication they could give me to ease or counteract this effect.

Before I could take the tests and scans at Bay City Medical Center, all
traces of the thyroid medication had to be removed from my system, as it
would camouflage further cancer symptoms. During these upcoming
tests, they would inject me with a radioactive iodine solution, and if there
were cancer cells or tumors in my body, this solution would be absorbed
by the thyroid tumor, which would show in the scan.

I had to be off my medication for at least three weeks prior to taking
these tests. The unpleasant withdrawal symptoms lasted all that time. It
would take about six weeks after going back on the medication before I
would begin to look and feel normal again.

All I really knew at this point was that a mistake had definitely been
made, and I was willing to believe it had been an honest one, if only the
people involved—namely, Kearny himself—would come forward and explain this to me, face to face.

I decided to contact Reverend Horace Williams, whom I had met through my activities with other cancer patients. I invited him to come to the house and see me. I was very ill and distraught at this time.

I was determined to give Dr. Kearny every opportunity to come forward and talk to me, as one fallible human being to another. So when I saw the minister, I asked him if he could arrange a meeting between Kearny and myself, with the minister also on hand to act as a witness or mediator. I told Williams the whole story that day, revealing my fears and suspicions about Kearny. However, when I related my story, I didn't mention the name of the doctor, though I felt sure Williams knew. He listened attentively while I told him my story. I could see he was visibly moved to hear what an ordeal I had been through.

When I finished the account, William's shoulders sagged and he was obviously saddened. "Tell me, Paula, is the doctor you're talking about Dr. Kearny?"

"Yes," I admitted, "it is."

It was then that I asked him to set up a meeting with Kearny. But he strongly advised against this. "No, Paula, do not confront Dr. Kearny with this. You've got to trust me. It would not be the right thing to do. Promise me you'll never go to him."

He seemed deadly serious about this, and I knew at once I had to trust his judgment, because he had known Kearny for many years. "Alright, I'll trust your advice," I told him. "Possibly you know more about this case than I do."

However, when I asked him why he felt I shouldn't confront Kearny with this, Williams refused to answer. "Maybe Kearny has already confided in you about this mixup," I said, "so probably this isn't the first time you've heard about it, though possibly he didn't mention my name. So now, for the first time, you know I'm the one involved."

He listened to all this, but he refused to acknowledge whether he agreed or disagreed. Perhaps, I thought, I was putting him in a delicate position wherein he might be betraying the confidence of others if he got personally involved in my situation.

Yet, I still wanted him to know how I felt. "I have a feeling Kearny has done this sort of thing to other patients, and if that is true, he must be stopped."

Solemnly, Reverend Williams again advised me against going to Kearny with this. "Promise me you won't try to go to him, Paula." I gave my promise.

"I'll grant you Dr. Kearny is a very strange man. Sometimes he says the strangest things," said Reverend Williams.

As it turned out, even though the minister was dead set against this idea, I felt better for having made this gesture. Now I could tell myself I had given Kearny every benefit of the doubt. But when I told Steve about this, he said, "Don't you ever do that again. And don't you ever consider confronting Kearny with this until we actually know what happened."

Nevertheless, I still felt I had fulfilled my obligation in making this attempt.

On May 14, 1979, Steve drove me up to Bay City for the three days of tests I would be given at the Center.

Following one of the scans at the Center, Dr. O'Brien, of the Nuclear Medicine Department, asked me, "Mrs. Carroll, who did your first thyroid surgery?"

"Dr. Jud Kearny."

"I see," he said. "And who did your second thyroid surgery?"

"Dr. Jeffrey Forbes."

"And does he also practice at the same hospital as Dr. Kearny?"

"Yes."

"Well, I hope you realize that Dr. Forbes saved your life." On the last day of my tests, Dr. O'Brien came running into my room looking very excited. They had just completed the bone scan.

"Oh, Mrs. Carroll," he said breathlessly, "we didn't find a tumor!"

What he was referring to here was that thyroid cancer will often metastasize into the bones or the lungs, which was what they were looking for. They were also concerned that the cancer had spread into my vocal chords. But not until they got the results of the body scan did they know for sure. Which explains Dr. O'Brien's excitement, as this was definitely good news and, I gathered, something of a surprise as well. But it wasn't until then that I realized this added possibility had existed, that the thyroid cancer could have metastasized to my bones or lungs.

When Steve and I saw Dr. Nicholson later that day, he said, "Mrs. Carroll, you are indeed fortunate. There is no doubt about it—you would not have survived with the residual cancer Dr. Kearny left."

I asked, "Is it possible Dr. Kearny didn't know he was leaving cancer?"

Looking down for a few moments, as if to ponder his answer, then looking straight at me with a determined expression, Dr. Nicholson said, "No, Mrs. Carroll. Dr. Kearny knew he was leaving cancer. He had the same information we had."

"Why would he deliberately withhold this vital information from us?" Steve asked.

"Well," Dr. Nicholson continued, "when Dr. Kearny realized he had surgically invaded the capsule of the tumor, he knew he had caused the cancer cells to spread into the bloodstream. The fact that your cancer was very well localized meant your chances for complete cure were eighty-five percent or better. Kearny knew his negligence had caused your cancer to become metastatic. I regret that I have to tell you these horrendous facts, Mr. and Mrs. Carroll, because you've had more than your share of bad news, but I truly believe that Dr. Kearny should be challenged. What he did is appalling.''

Now we knew how serious my case was. Of course, Steve and I were stunned to hear the dismal truth. But, again, there was a feeling of relief at finally learning the facts of what had happened one and a half years earlier.

I had been carrying a heavy burden of guilt during this period, thinking that in some way I was to blame for all that was happening to me. I now see that this was a truly irrational assumption, in view of how I was victimized by others. Still, that's how I felt at the time.

It was also during this same crisis point that I finally came to the conclusion that the guilt I carried was not my own. When I was finally able to face and accept this reality, I began to rebuild my self-respect. I now believed that none of this had been my fault, that I had been treated carelessly and unprofessionally at every step.

While I was at the Center, I was also given a therapeutic dosage of radioactive iodine to treat my metastatic thyroid cancer. Dr. Nicholson told me, ''If the treatment is not successful, it would be too great a risk to leave it.'' He was referring to the residual thyroid tissue they had found in the scan. So I was scheduled to return to the Center in August. If the ablation treatment was not successful, I would need more surgery at that time.

Although going back on my thyroid medication proved to be another difficult transition, it was like heaven to be told I could resume taking this medication. While I'm on it, I feel normal, meaning I can function normally. And naturally, I eventually returned to my normal weight and appearance.

Finally, my tests and scans were completed, and Steve arrived to drive me back home. He was in a joyful, emotional mood because I hadn't been given a terminal prognosis, after all. Steve took heart in knowing the happy outcome of O'Brien's scans, and despite my remaining fears and uncertainties, I supported his need to rejoice while we drove home that day.

Up until that point, he and I had been through an unending period of anguish and worry. For us, this had been a real nightmare, like something we never could have anticipated happening to us. We had always planned everything so carefully, worked so hard for what we had—who could have expected such an outlandish series of crises? Neither of us had been ready for the ordeal we had faced, so now we had reason to hope again, and it felt good.

Chapter Eleven

*N*ot long after I returned from my tests in Bay City, in late May of 1979, Steve and I felt we had no other recourse but to go through more formal channels to rectify the great wrongs done to me. We began discussing the idea of pursuing some sort of investigation, though first we knew we would need some documentary evidence to back us up.

I now learned that the two letters from the Mayo Clinic were at the pathology lab. The letters were from Dr. Morgan Baker, of the Mayo Clinic. One of them was dated January, 1978, and the other was dated March, 1979. Steve and I went to the lab to get copies of the letters.

The January, 1978 letter was one of the letters which Kearny had withheld from my records when I transferred to Dr. Melvin Henderman. Of course, I didn't realize those letters would be at the pathology lab until I phoned and spoke to my friend, Miriam Powell, the lady who had cut new slides and sent them up to Dr. Nicholson earlier. She inadvertently told me that the letters from the Mayo Clinic were there.

When we arrived at the lab, I asked her for copies of the letters.

"Well, Paula, copies have been given to Dr. Forbes, so he has all the information, and he knows what happened."

"Please Miriam, I want copies of the letters," I said firmly.

She stammered around a bit, obviously surprised that I would pursue this, finally asking, "Well, why do you want them?"

"Steve and I want to review them ourselves."

She told us Dr. Forbes had them and we could look at his copies. "We want our own copies. There's no reason we have to ask Dr. Forbes to see his." I concluded by saying she should make up the copies, and Steve would be back later to pick them up.

At long last I was being firm. Steve went back an hour later and picked them up. Then he and I sat down and tried to decipher what had actually been said in these letters. But we found Miriam had tried to side-track us a little: she only gave Steve the letter of March, 1979, and had withheld the other letter. So I sent Steve right back for the missing letter, advising Miriam by phone that he was on his way for the "rest of the information." She made a copy of the missing letter and had it ready for Steve to pick up.

We read the letter of January, 1978 first, in which it stated, ". . . *if* the surgical margin of resection did not contain tumor. . . ." But we knew that Dr. Nicholson and his pathologist, Dr. Moss, had found that the surgical margins *did* contain tumor. Knowing this, wouldn't that single statement from Mayo's Dr. Baker be enough to alert Dr. Kearny to check out the possibility?

In the March, 1979 letter, Dr. Baker said he found the residual papillary carcinoma embedded in scar tissue from the previous excisional biopsy. Obviously, Dr. Kearny was afraid to take any corrective steps at this time for fear his original blunder would be revealed. That's why he didn't take blood tests, and also why he refused to do the customary follow-ups or any thyroid scans after my surgery. He didn't want any documentation of his incompetence. All his negligence was designed to cover up that first blunder. It was obvious that the only thing that mattered to Kearny was his reputation.

After Steve and I read those letters, I said, "Steve, the fact they're saying 'if' the surgical margins of resection didn't contain tumor . . . that means Mayo didn't see the surgical margins when they sent that specimen back in January of 1978. Why didn't the pathology lab send Mayo those surgical margins?"

Steve agreed this was a good question, though as yet, neither of us had a good answer—to anything. However, obtaining those two letters gave us enough information to substantiate our rising suspicions.

Interestingly enough, the new slides Miriam Powell made and sent up to Dr. Nicholson had *included* the margins. She apparently did this on her own, though I have a feeling she was in trouble after it was revealed what she had done. She sent them up to Nicholson and Moss so they could see the invasion of the tumor. Why Miriam did this, I'm not sure. Because the previous slides had not included the margins, Miriam had, without realizing it, implicated the pathology lab.

Now, of course, so many "mysteries" have become clear to me. Kearny deliberately lied to convince me he had done more extensive surgery than a mere biopsy. That in itself was a criminal act, insofar as he was lying about a situation that involved a potentially terminal illness and could, indeed, help it to become terminal by his very actions. I was now convinced that Kearny knew at the time that he *had* invaded the capsule of the tumor during surgery. I realized I was right to suspect both Post and Kearny of a coverup, as it was now clear they had both lied to me repeatedly.

However, I don't believe Dr. Forbes realized that Dr. Post was so involved in my case, though he had to know Post assisted with my first thyroid surgery. Still, I feel Forbes thought he could simply isolate Kearny and get to him alone. But in doing so, Forbes didn't realize that the entire Tissue Committee had entered into the coverup when the surgery report did not match up with the specimen—the thyroid specimen of January, 1978—and they could see that the tumor had been invaded. They could also see cancer on the surgical margins. Both Post and Kearny were on the Tissue Committee at that time.

From experience regarding the mishandling of other cases, the pathology lab knew what Kearny was doing, knew what he was capable of. The pathologists wrote on my tissue report that I'd had a total right lobectomy when they knew I had not. So they were in on the coverup as well. They knew that I'd only had a biopsy from Kearny. In fact, it was called a nodulectomy, because all Kearny really did was to excise the nodule. He had told me this the day after the surgery.

Furthermore, the pathology lab deliberately sent only the slides of the tumor to Mayo Clinic, and not the surgical margins, following the January, 1978 surgery, because they didn't want Mayo to see that the surgical margins *did* contain cancer. This was their part of the coverup, and as such, it was a criminal act to withhold such vital information. Those in the lab had carefully selected just the slides that would show Mayo the tumor, but not the margins. This incriminating evidence documented the criminal conspiracy that existed between Kearny and the pathology lab doctors.

Remember, the letter from Mayo Clinic had stated, *"if"* the surgical margins did not contain tumor, which proves those margins had not been sent but had been deliberately withheld, because those in the pathology lab didn't want Mayo to see them, as it would show that the cancerous tumor had been invaded. In other words, it would have revealed the Big Foul-up.

They were all getting together to protect the noblest blunderer of them all—Jud Kearny. I suppose one had to hand it to him for being enormously popular among his peers. But one must wonder what kind of power this man had to rally such support.

In any case, when the pathology lab sent the second specimen to the Mayo Clinic, as requested by Dr. Forbes, following my second thyroid surgery in March of 1979, they again sent only the slides which did *not* contain residual cancer. Or at least, that had been their original plan. Actually, it was such a waste even to consider sending all that inaccurate material, knowing that Mayo couldn't have responded with an accurate report. It was just part of the elaborate scam all of these medical professionals were into, preserving the big fiction, and thus creating a true obstruction of medical justice.

Ironically enough, these people were ultimately caught up in their own incompetency: in one of the slides sent to Mayo, the pathology lab had not seen the residual cancer, so they inadvertently sent some incriminating evidence to the Mayo Clinic. As a result, at least part of the truth got out in spite of their efforts, which proves these amateurs couldn't even handle their own coverup successfully. When Mayo detected this bit of evidence they sent the letter that shook Forbes up so badly as he read it aloud to me in his office that day.

And too, at this time, I was able to piece together a rather accurate impression of just what I felt had gone on at that hospital staff meeting which was held at the time of my second thyroid surgery. I think that when Dr. Forbes discovered how Kearny had messed up my original thyroid surgery and left me to die, he misjudged the extent of the coverup. I also believe that Forbes thought we would never find out the truth because of the garbled facts.

So, at this point, I feel Dr. Forbes was beset by a lot of tension and inner conflicts. On the one hand, he was truly worried about my condition, while on the other, he feared for his own culpability, knowing he had gotten into this conspiracy way over his head.

After Steve and I read those two incriminating letters from Mayo Clinic, we paid a visit to Dr. Forbes. Steve talked to Forbes about the various procedures involved in my treatment, asking the doctor certain leading questions that were obviously making him tense and nervous. Finally, Steve asked him: "How does residual cancer become embedded in scar tissue?"

Looking down at the floor, Forbes answered, "I don't know." For once our questions weren't answered with an evasion; this was an outright lie.

During that visit Forbes asked me how I was doing after resuming my thyroid medication. I told him I hadn't been feeling very well.

With that, Forbes stared at me and blurted out, "Well, you're finally going to admit you're human. Huh." That exasperated me, as I knew exactly what he was implying: they had all been wondering when I was going to break down and complain and actually admit I felt lousy. And yet these doctors hate having to deal with chronic complainers for patients. Moreover, for some time they had all known a lot more about my symptoms than I did.

Forbes continued to be tense and evasive all during that meeting, until finally Steve and I realized he wasn't about to answer any of our direct questions truthfully. By now it was clear to us that the medical Mafia had "gotten" to Dr. Jeffrey Forbes.

While all this was going on, I still found time to involve myself with the Hospice Movement; my work here continued to be very fulfilling. Counseling other cancer patients did not add to my own depression, for I thought only of the contribution I was making by simply keeping them company at a time like that. I clearly saw their desperate need, their isolation and loneliness. So often people are afraid to directly confront those who might be terminal. I had as many as eight cancer patients to counsel at a time, so it was a very rewarding project for me, one which I managed to continue through June of 1979.

Yet during this time, I was soon wondering where I could go for such counseling, because, as I've mentioned, I received no such therapy after any of my various surgeries. I was still shocked after learning the dreadful truth about Dr. Kearny. I was also disillusioned and hurt to think that a man whom I trusted so implicitly could have knowingly made such a serious error without making any efforts to correct the damage later. And when I realized how many others knew of his blunder but had agreed to keep it quiet, I was broken-hearted to think these men were, in fact, willing to let me die.

It seemed so ironic to remember how well I had handled my surgical and medical crises, compared with how ill-equipped I was to cope with this massive betrayal. I needed someone to confide in about all this, though I still refused to share these problems with Steve or any members of my family, because I knew how it would distress them. Luckily, I remembered a friend of mine in town who is also a counselor, Harriet Monroe. I called her and began seeing her on a regular basis, confiding in her, literally pouring my heart out to her as I told her what an ordeal I had been put through at the hands of Drs. Kearny, Post, and Forbes.

In time, Harriet became my one and only confidante and my dearest friend. She provided the kind of comfort and understanding I had needed for so long; she was a compassionate listener, someone I wasn't afraid to go to with the truth, someone I knew I could trust. It was such a release for me to get all these feelings out into the open, and Harriet never failed to be perceptive and sympathetic. She gave me the kind of courage I needed to face the many challenges that still lay ahead of me.

Steve and I went to a party one evening in early June, and once again we ran into Dr. Kearny and his wife. Throughout this period I kept running into this man, quite by accident, at the oddest times. I thought how difficult it had been to get in to see him, thanks to Mrs. Sumner's interference, and now when he was the last person on earth I wanted to look at, I was practically tripping over him everywhere I went.

Nevertheless, I was cordial to Kearny and his wife. I walked up to Mrs. Kearny, shook her hand and said, "Good evening, Norma, how are you?"

I then stepped forward and shook Dr. Kearny's hand. Trying to maintain his composure, he said, "Paula! It's so good to see you. . . ." He patted me on the shoulder.

It was during that month of June that Steve and I also talked seriously about launching an official investigation, though I was still somewhat reluctant, because I didn't want to jeopardize my position as Dr. Forbes's patient. After all, where on earth could I go for treatment if all the doctors in town suddenly refused to see me? Nevertheless, Steve and I both agreed it was our moral responsibility to challenge the wrong that had been perpetrated against me, for fear that this same thing had happened to others and would continue unless someone stopped it.

In order to try and discourage us from the type of challenge that Steve and I were contemplating, a nurse friend related this story to me about a doctor. He proudly declared at a medical meeting, "We have this town sewed up. If anyone tries to sue us we'll hear about it. They won't stand a chance." Armed with this knowledge, our first decision regarding a lawyer was to look for one out of town, as far away from our own section of the state as we could get. We chose an attorney by the name of Harry Claxton in a distant community. Steve and I shared with him what Dr. Nicholson had told us. After we discussed our case, he said, "There's one thing missing in your case."

"And what is that?" I asked him.

"You didn't die," he replied. "If you had died your estate would have had a great case."

I wondered if that was my cue to apologize. Or perhaps I should have said, "Well, nobody's perfect!" He had actually implied that as a corpse, I could really prove damages.

Back in March of 1978, when I took my records out of town to Dr. Henderman, Steve and I had opened them up and made copies of all of them. That was how I later knew that certain records were missing. Mr.

Claxton pointed out that the surgical record did not coincide with what the pathology report had said about the same specimen that was removed, which proved there was a marked discrepancy between the surgical report and the pathology report.

Mr. Claxton felt that indicated there was sufficient evidence that important information had been deliberately concealed and agreed to investigate. He then told us he would subpoena my records. He would do this through a microfilm company in San Jose that specializes in microfilming records in doctors' offices. The doctors are compelled to let them do this, as the company has subpoena powers.

However, it would be awhile before Harry Claxton got around to doing this, as he turned out to be quite a slow mover. But because I had a post-op visit with Dr. Forbes coming up in three weeks, I instructed Claxton to take no action at all until I had had this vital checkup. I wanted to tell Forbes about the investigation because I didn't want to spring any surprises.

During that visit to Dr. Forbes's office in mid-July, I told him frankly that there would be an investigation. But that was all I said; I mentioned nothing about a lawsuit.

But as soon as I uttered the word "investigation," Forbes quickly asked me, "Are you going to sue?"

After he said that, I grew very tense, wondering if Forbes would now refuse to treat me. To answer his question, I said something evasive, wanting to put him off, knowing how much I needed at least one doctor in town. But instead of acting defensive or suspicious, Forbes took me completely by surprise. He came over to me, gave me a big hug and said, "You know how I feel about you, Paula. You're the kind of patient that makes me proud I'm a doctor, and makes it worthwhile to get up in the morning and come to work. I hope you won't sue." Then he left the room.

When I recovered from my surprise, I reviewed what he had actually said. In essence, his message was: "I love you like a sister, so don't sue me." Yet, at this point we had only instructed our attorney to obtain my records. Now, however, Forbes's quick mention of a lawsuit convinced me we had good reason to demand those records. I also felt that Forbes had been telling me he felt I had a reason to sue, so perhaps, in a way, he really hoped I would.

In late July, just before I was due to go back to the Center for more tests, the Hospice group did several newspaper articles about cancer patients, to be serialized in the local paper. I was called and asked if I would be interviewed. I agreed, provided my name would be kept out of the paper. They agreed to quote me but not use my name. Naturally, during the course of the interview, I mentioned nothing about the medical inequities I'd been involved in; nothing about my case at all.

I spoke to the reporter about my readjustment, my surgery—mentioning no doctors' names—and my personal adjustments to the ailment, stressing how important it was for each patient to build themselves a strong support system in dealing with the emotional and physical aftermath of such surgery.

Meanwhile, aside from the legal aspects of this case, I also had some medical problems to contend with. At the end of July I had to go off my thyroid medication again to prepare for more scans and tests I would undergo at Bay City Medical Center in August. That meant I would now face the same torturous symptoms all over again. But at the Center I was convinced I was in the right hands, so I faced this new hurdle with a lot more hope than fear.

Chapter Twelve

$\mathcal{M}$y new tests were to take several days, from August 5th through the 9th.

As my breast and thyroid cancers are not connected, tests can only be done for one of these ailments at a time. This makes it rather difficult, because while I'm having thyroid tests, any other tests pertaining to my breast cancer must be delayed. This is due to the fact that my body can only tolerate a certain amount of these debilitating tests at one time. A long interval must come between these tests, to give me a chance to recuperate.

As yet, I hadn't had any tests for my breast cancer. They'd had to put off doing that while I was undergoing the thyroid tests. Dr. Nicholson had said that "there was no doubt" that my own persistence saved my life. To realize how close I came to having my condition become irreversible was disturbing.

During that summer, I read an article in our local paper which, for the first time, acquainted me with the state Medical Standards Board— usually referred to as MSB. It wasn't surprising that I hadn't heard about this agency, as it was only organized in 1975. I now learned that it was a doctor-monitoring system created to assure the patient of competent medical care.

It was now possible, I read—and indeed, it was recommended—that unethical doctors be reported to this board in order to have the proper action instigated.

The disciplinary action taken against the offending doctors would vary, I learned, from a short probationary period to revocation of the doctor's license, depending on the nature of the offense.

I called this agency the next morning, and asked them several questions. Specifically, I asked them if there had been any complaints filed against Dr. Jud Kearny. Their response was immediate. On the phone they told me, from memory, without looking it up, that there had been a report filed against him, but it was so lengthy they would send me a copy in the mail.

I was more shocked than ever to realize I was not the only trusting patient he had harmed. This also meant quite conclusively that I had *not* been imagining things after all; that despite all his surface charm, and his grand, paternal manner, Kearny was a seasoned bungler.

The clerk to whom I spoke said that once an accusation is filed and there's been a hearing, this information then becomes public record. When I received the copy of the hearing, I was further appalled. Kearny was under some kind of disciplinary action, and was being closely monitored by MSB.

It was also in this report that I learned something even more dreadful about Kearny. In 1973, while performing varicose vein surgery on a man, he had stripped the femoral artery instead of the saphenous vein. As a result, three days later the patient's leg had to be amputated. I was horrified to read this, and to think the doctor who had done this was still free to perform his incompetent surgeries.

When I spoke about this to the investigator with MSB, he told me the victim in this case still didn't know the truth, or that his leg had been amputated needlessly only because of Kearny's careless blunder. It was even more difficult to believe that Dr. Forbes, still the only local doctor I thought I could trust, had testified in Kearny's behalf, along with five other doctors, during the hearing. However, I later learned the kind of pressure Kearny exerted against Forbes and the others to insure their support.

Apparently, neither the amputee nor his family ever launched a suit against Kearny, as they never knew what had happened. And yet it was later reported to the MSB, because whenever there is an insurance settlement of thirty thousand dollars or more, it is a state law that it has to be reported by the insurance company.[1]

After the victim's leg was amputated, the insurance adjuster went to see him while he was still in the hospital and told him, ''It was an unfortunate complication, and there will be a settlement.''

Once again, it was a case of the experts relying on the ignorance of the laymen, i.e., their patients. And in this case, the insurance company moved in very fast to hush the patient up with a quick offer of a cash settlement. This was because Kearny had been sued for malpractice so many times before, the insurance company knew it would be difficult to defend him in court. This further confirmed what I had already learned, that the average citizen automatically trusts his doctor, usually without question. And when, as in my case, they finally learn the nature of the offense, it's almost impossible to prove an injury that is done in such a covert situation, within the confines of the surgeon's operating room where all the "witnesses" are other doctors or medical personnel and thus, sworn to secrecy.

In the case of the patient who needlessly lost his leg there was a hearing, conducted by the MSB, and the victim was told about the hearing in advance, though he was never told the exact charge against Dr. Kearny. During the hearing the injured patient was deliberately taken into an outer room, away from the proceedings. There he was asked by one of the investigators: "If you were to have this same surgery now, would you return to Dr. Kearny?"

He said, "Yes, I suppose so." Obviously, he had no idea what Kearny had done to him, and no one had seen fit to tell him the nature of the hearing against the doctor. Once again, the combination of ignorance and blind trust was on Kearny's side. Oddly enough, the victim didn't even connect this investigation with his amputation. Yet the fact that he was there at all should at least have given him a hint that there was, in fact, a very real connection. On the other hand, at that point it was probably best he wasn't told all the horrible facts, as there was no action he could have taken after the official hearing, and after he had already accepted the insurance settlement. Of course, by not telling him the truth, the insurance company saved themselves a great deal of money.

This further proves how certain doctors rely on the general ignorance of their patients to protect them whenever they commit medical malpractice. In fact, many patients never detect malpractice until it's too late and the "complication" has already proven fatal.

I now realized what the attorney had meant when he said I would have a much stronger case if Kearny's foul-up had killed me. It also occurred to me that in most such cases, it is usually left to the heirs to take any action *if* they are aware of the true facts. This, of course, made me newly thankful that I was still alive and strong enough to initiate this corrective action on my own.

As for the ultimate findings of the MSB hearing against Kearny, the Review Committee admonished him as follows: "It is strongly recommended that respondent dictate his operating reports immediately after surgery, and that all of his notes and reports contain a complete record of relevant findings regarding patient care and treatment, including complete results of physical examinations of patients." During the hearing he had feigned a poor memory due to incomplete records. This excuse had worked effectively for him on previous malpractice cases. Why shouldn't this same scheme work again? Actually, I saw the admonishment as an elaborate "slap on the wrist," not nearly a strong enough deterrent, even though it was clear they now meant to monitor Dr. Kearny.

We were later told by one of the MSB investigators that they felt they had an open-and-shut case against Kearny, that normally the MSB does not take such action against a doctor unless he is a chronic incompetent, and further, a single complaint against a doctor will rarely ever result in a hearing. The investigator also told us that because of an inexperienced judge, the only one in the panel of six who refused to vote against Kearny, MSB lost the case.

However, the fact that he now knew he was going to be monitored only made him that much more proficient as a liar and a coverup artist. Now he had more incentive to go underground and become more devious, as he was still more strongly motivated to cover up his mistakes instead of learning how not to repeat them.

It is hard to believe that it didn't bother this man to realize he was obviously no longer in possession of his skills. If he had ever been a dedicated surgeon, he would have been the first to observe his waning abilities, and he should have been the one to cease further surgery. Knowing what he might do to another surgical patient should have stopped him at that point, voluntarily. That would also have been far smarter than waiting for lawsuits and unfavorable publicity to start circulating. But with Kearny, it was clear that his ego and vanity kept him from stepping down off his pedestal.

If Kearny were really the fine and honorable citizen he pretended to be, and was believed to be, he would have done the noble thing. Knowing he might end up killing some innocent patient, he should have willingly turned in his knife.

When we learned of these new disclosures, Steve and I were appalled to think that the man to whom we were both willing to give "the benefit of the doubt" had turned out to be even worse than we could have imagined. This man had become so obsessed with his image, he didn't care about the human lives he was jeopardizing—his main concern was to preserve his public reputation.

Now I shudder to recall how completely I had trusted this man—to the extent that I had actually placed my life in his hands. But it seemed even more outrageous that he should be permitted to go on committing his surgical atrocities on other innocent patients. It was my fervent hope to prevent that from happening. This strengthened my determination to stop Kearny and to expose the conspiracy he and his colleagues had instigated. But most important of all, I wanted to make sure this never happened to anyone else. I now saw this as my true moral obligation in this case. I did a great deal of soul searching, and consulted with several ministers who strongly advised me to pursue a legal course.

If I were to do nothing, I would be compromising, I would be giving my silent approval to the misdeeds of others. I certainly did not want to confront this dishonesty—I would much rather someone else did it. But I could also see that as I was the one who perceived this wrongdoing, for me to do nothing would mean I was voting for wrong. Too many people think that standing up to wrong and challenging it won't bring their loved ones back. This attitude is the epitome of selfishness, because they are admitting that they won't try to change the system for the benefit of others.

On September 13th our attorney finally sent the microfilm company to Dr. Kearny's office to film my records. They had notified him about this visit in advance by sending him a card, which he returned, giving them his permission. Of course, knowing in advance that they meant to film the records meant Kearny had ample time to withhold whatever he wanted.

Nevertheless, when the company representative arrived in his office, Kearny flatly refused to give them permission to film. Instead, he gave him a set of records which he himself had copied, telling the man the records were complete. He signed a certificate, under penalty of perjury, saying that the copies were true and complete. This, of course, turned out to be untrue.

When Steve and I reviewed the records, we found that the October 13, 1977 surgical report was missing. There were several other discrepancies as well, which led us to believe there were two sets of records. Also, the January 13, 1978 surgical report in the folder given to the microfilm company showed that Dr. Butler did a frozen section, and this report was *not* signed by Kearny. (As I've mentioned, Steve and I had earlier made our own copies of the original report, which enabled us to match them up and uncover the discrepancies.) The January 13, 1978 surgical report Kearny had given to Dr. Henderman—the same report Steve and I had copied while we had the records in our possession (this was also the copy Kearny filed)—stated that a Dr. Neeley did the frozen section, and it *was* signed by Kearny.

The microfilm company later told us they'd been in business for over thirty years, and this was the first time a doctor had ever refused them permission to film medical records. Surely, we thought, that in itself was at least a hint of an admission of guilt on Kearny's part. Although they'd had a court order, they didn't want to press the issue at that point, so they accepted the copies Kearny gave them.

A few days later I received a call from the receptionist in Dr. Nicholson's Bay City office. She told me that a man had been there to microfilm my records. She wanted to know if I was suing and if so, why?

As briefly as I could, I brought her up to date on the whole hideous story, certain from her shocked reaction that this was the first she had heard about it. She said, "All I knew, Mrs. Carroll, was the very serious condition you were in when you first came to us. But I thought the doctor who sent you here was the one who did your first surgery. My goodness, you sure have every right to sue."

On September 18th, I kept an appointment with Dr. Forbes to have a routine post-op checkup. I felt slightly uneasy about going to him, knowing that only five days earlier the microfilm people had been to his office to film *his* records. Naturally his attitude was quite changed. No loving "big brother" act this time. Instead, he was very reserved and sarcastic. Of course, by now he knew of our legal investigation, so I really didn't expect him to act any differently than he did.

At this point, however, I had to conclude that this sort of unpopularity would come with the territory. And the fact remained: it was purely academic whether or not I treated these men like enemies; they had been treating me as their enemy for a long time now.

During that month I continued going to the public library to study various medical books in an effort to understand what had really happened to me.

One day I ran into an old friend at the library, Penelope Beaumont, the wife of a local physician. She wanted to know why I was doing all that medical research. So I briefly told her what had happened to me, though without mentioning the doctor's name. She was horrified.

"Oh, Paula!" she exclaimed. "That sounds like a nightmare!"

"It is," I said simply.

By now Steve had joined me in this diligent research, and we continued to study and investigate on our own, trying to make some logical sense of the records. This was a very tedious and confusing time for both of us. Sometimes I would have sleepless nights, when I would get up, go into the dining room in the darkness, and sit on the floor with my back to the wall and pray. It was so difficult to understand why this had happened, and why these doctors had treated me with such contempt. I was literally grieved.

Ironically enough, it was about this time that one of my friends said,

"You know, Paula, your trouble is that nobody believes how sick you've been, because you never *look* sick; you just keep looking so healthy and vivacious." I couldn't see it as a problem that outside I didn't reflect what was falling apart inside, though it was rather consoling to know I still had my looks. If I had gone around with a long face, I would have been accused of trying to extract every bit of sympathy from my situation. I had to learn to live with these two attitudinal extremes: either you're not sick at all, or you're about to die.

By December of 1979, Steve and I became disenchanted with Harry Claxton, our attorney. Although he had obtained our records, he hadn't done anything with them in all this time. We kept waiting for him to do something constructive, until finally we decided he was moving too slowly for us. We got busy and found another lawyer in a distant city, as we still wanted to stay comfortably away from our own town.

Our new lawyer was a wiry, cross-eyed, dark-haired man by the name of Floyd Lawrence. We ended up calling him Flaky Floyd, however, because of a few erratic decisions he made in our case.

We brought him copies of the records and told him of our case. He said what Kearny had done to me was despicable, and continued, "You definitely have a legitimate complaint, and I agree that man shouldn't be allowed to practice medicine." We also presented proof of the coverup and conspiracy.

There is a law which proclaims that anyone suing a doctor for medical malpractice must send a ninety-day notice informing the doctor of that intention. Our first lawyer had neglected to do this, though we later learned he was heavily involved with another huge lawsuit at the time, which had distracted him from our case. I was worried that the statute of limitations would run out, which would have happened on December 18th. But now that we had it on record that our ninety-day notice had been sent, that would automatically give us another ninety days. (Incidentally, anyone who wants to sue for malpractice in our state must do so no later than one year after the date of discovery of the injury.)

Claxton had also mistakenly told us we had until March before our time ran out, but our new lawyer knew at once that we didn't have that much time, so we got faster action from him. We realized that Dr. Kearny had to know of this statute of limitations; thus, he must have felt that the longer this went on undiscovered, the safer he would be. Consequently, I feel we made a wise move in finding an attorney who would expedite these proceedings for us. This now meant we would get our action in right under the wire.

On the day the notices were served, Dr. Post called Steve and demanded to know why we were suing him. "You were the assisting surgeon and we want your testimony," Steve told him.

Post vehemently professed his innocence. "Believe me, Steve, I had no idea what happened, that Dr. Kearny left part of the tumor. You must understand I wasn't involved with any of that. . . !" He went on and on with a lot of evasive double-talk, desperate to get off the hook. But Steve wasn't buying this story.

It was also at this time that I decided to go directly to the state's Medical Standards Board and personally sign an accusation against Dr. Kearny. I was told this was a very unusual action for a patient to take, but I knew that the court case could be held up for five years, and I felt that Dr. Kearny must be stopped.

---

[1] *West's Annotated California Code, Business and Professions Code*, § 2231. Repealed by Stats.1982, c. 823, p. 3128, § 5.5. This statute, enacted in 1980 (Stats.1980, c. 1313, p. 4473, 2.), was repealed in 1982 as noted above. The text of this statute follows:

The circumstances of practice of any licensee shall be investigated where there have been any judgments, settlements, or arbitration awards requiring the licensee or the licencee's professional liability insurer to pay an amount in damages in excess of a cumulative total of thirty thousand dollars ($30,000) with respect to any claim that injury or damage was proximately caused by the licensee's error, negligence, or omission.

Chapter Thirteen

On December 12th, I received an anonymous mailing of an article that had been copied from a medical magazine known as *Cancer News*. The article was entitled, "Doctor, Doctor, Cut My Throat," written by Isaac Asimov, the well-known science fiction writer, though he is definitely no medical expert.

It was a frivolous and very unscientific discussion of thyroid cancer which downgraded the seriousness of the disease in a most unprofessional manner. An article like this demonstrates the ignorance surrounding thyroid cancer, even among some doctors. While it is true that thyroid cancer has a high rate of cure, that's only because the tumor tends to stay well encapsulated. But when the patient is in the hands of an incompetent, deceitful surgeon who cuts into the tumor and knowingly leaves a part of it, the cancer is spread. In my case, if Dr. Kearny had performed the surgery correctly in the first place, I would never have needed the second surgery or the many tests and follow-up treatments that came afterwards. To know that all that additional anguish was caused by one man's failure to be honest makes his medical incompetence even more heinous.

Naturally I was very upset when I read that article. I didn't even tell Steve about it. I checked with the library and learned that only doctors receive this technical magazine, which told me it must have come from a local doctor. It was a cruel and vicious trick to play on someone who'd had two thyroid surgeries and countless tests and scans. The fact that I probably knew someone mentally deranged and callous enough to do this was disturbing.

During the early part of January, 1980, I had occasion to visit several friends of mine who were patients at the hospital, and one day I ran into Dr. Forbes. I gave him my usual friendly greeting, but he just looked at me with a cold and icy glare and barely spoke. It was obvious he had heard that I had filed a complaint directly with MSB. But, I thought, this shouldn't concern him; he's not involved in this complaint.

Later that month I kept an appointment for a check-up with Dr. Nicholson in Bay City. He found another lump in the neck area. He said he would contact Dr. Forbes and get him to perform a biopsy.

A few days after I had seen Dr. Nicholson, at a time when I thought our legal action was progressing nicely, I was astonished to receive a letter from our lawyer, Floyd Lawrence. He wrote that he'd had a doctor review my records, after which this doctor recommended that I sue Drs. Forbes and Nicholson. He went on to state that I had no case against Dr. Kearny, as, in his opinion, Kearny had done the right thing during my thyroid treatment.

I was stunned by this development. I couldn't comprehend how any doctor could read all those incriminating records and still conclude that we had no case against Kearny. Yet in his letter, Lawrence implied this doctor claimed Kearny had done the right thing during the thyroid surgery.

Both the Mayo Clinic and the Bay City Medical Center agreed that Kearny had fouled up in my case, though, of course, both those clinics were far removed from us. We had taken it for granted we could trust our attorney without worrying that he would also be dragged into this conspiracy.

Steve and I thought this through and decided they were deliberately setting up a smoke screen in order to confuse and divert us. Originally, as Lawrence well knew, we only planned to sue Kearny, Post, and the hospital. But now, hoping to throw obstacles in our way to keep from getting anywhere with our legal action, they were trying to shift our attention to Drs. Nicholson and Forbes, the two men who had saved my life. Lawrence knew we never planned to take action against Forbes and Nicholson. We concluded this had to be a delaying tactic, a deliberate contrivance to waste precious time.

Now, of course, "Flaky" Floyd Lawrence informed us he couldn't possibly continue to represent us, because his friend had declared that we had no case against Kearny. By then I already suspected Lawrence's part in the coverup, so I wasn't all that shattered when he dumped us. Actually, Lawrence was blatantly contradicting himself here, having told us we should sue Forbes and Nicholson, while refusing to go on representing us because, ostensibly, we had no case against Kearny. Lawrence said the only real complaint I might have against Kearny was ". . . hurt feelings, and you can't sue for hurt feelings."

So if, as he wanted us to believe, we had a case against Forbes and Nicholson, why did he now refuse to represent us in that action? Lawrence knew as well as we did that we had no case against them. It was that little "sin of omission" that told us both Lawrence and his doctor friend had been induced to join the big coverup, probably at the request, and/or insistence, of Dr. Post. This, we felt, was another diversion tactic, designed to confuse, befuddle, and delay us.

Actually, the plot had now become so involved and nefarious, it was getting downright Shakespearean. But at least we knew very quickly what they were doing, and why. Meanwhile, "Flaky" Lawrence sent me a refund of what was left of our deposit fee.

By this time, however, we had no doubts that we had compiled strong and irrefutable evidence against Dr. Kearny, though it took months of research and investigation before we had ironclad proof, which didn't happen until the latter part of May, 1979. It reached the point where we actually had to put ten records together to compare and discover exactly what Kearny had done—it had been that cleverly hidden and falsified.

The day after I got Lawrence's outrageous letter, I received a phone call from a woman who really castigated me for having the nerve to sue such "a fine, upstanding man" as Dr. Kearny. She reminded me of the Bible verse, "One Christian must not sue another."

In reply, I told her, "The Apostle Paul wasn't talking about serious matters in that context, he was only discussing trivial acts." I felt it ironic that I was being severely criticized for suing the noble Jud Kearny when, at the very moment of her call, I didn't even have a lawyer!

Meanwhile, Steve was so infuriated by Lawrence's surprise betrayal that he drove to the attorney's office and told him what a cowardly thing he had done, to give up so easily when he knew perfectly well what a strong case we had. Oddly enough, Lawrence didn't attempt to argue this point; he even readily admitted it. And because we knew time was running out, we feared we wouldn't find another attorney in time to meet the deadline. That meant we were stuck with "Flaky" Lawrence, whether we trusted him or not. At the moment, taking time out to find an honest lawyer was a luxury we couldn't afford.

During the confrontation, Steve convinced Lawrence to hold tight and do nothing for the time being, while we compiled additional proof of the coverup and injury. So they left it like that: Lawrence agreed to go on representing us, but he would take no further action until he heard from us.

Earlier that week, I phoned Dr. Nicholson to make sure he had contacted Dr. Forbes to arrange for him to biopsy the lump Nicholson had found. I had particularly wanted Nicholson to intercede for me here, as I feared—in fact I had reason to know—that Forbes would be more than a little hostile towards me after the cold way he had treated me when I passed him in the hall at the hospital. Though I had terrible misgivings about the way this confrontation would turn out, I reminded myself that it was Forbes's second thyroid surgery that had literally saved my life. I could only hope he would remember that now also, and in view of what he now had to know about Kearny's involvement in this case, I hoped those factors would help to sustain this man's loyalty.

In any case, Nicholson confirmed that my appointment with Dr. Forbes had been made, and I kept that appointment later that week on January 30, 1980. I had good reason to worry about this new complication, as Nicholson had earlier phoned me to say, "You have a nodule in the right neck area." In the midst of my legal pressures, I was still beset by medical emergencies.

When I saw Forbes that day, he seemed friendly and relaxed—at first. He sat me on his stool so he could more easily palpate the neck area. As he did, he asked me, "How's the lawsuit coming, Paula?"

"I don't think I should discuss that with you," I said.

That made him angry, and rather surprised, too, to hear such a firm comeback from me. I went on, "I don't want to involve you any more than you already are."

"Yes, Paula, you should have that nodule biopsied, but I am not going to do it," he said with a smirk on his face. "When I talked with Dr. Nicholson I told him you would have to have the biopsy done in Bay City. Dr. Nicholson has a toehold up there. As a matter of fact, as long as you persist with this investigation you will never again receive medical treatment in this town."

I couldn't believe what I was hearing. This was the doctor who promised never to abandon me, and now he was doing it.

I said, "Okay, I understand. I cannot stop this investigation because what you doctors are doing is wrong. If I were to remain silent I would be approving of what I know is happening here. I cannot do that. You are asking me to compromise. Do what you must do, but I will not stop. Truth is on my side and that is a powerful weapon."

"Paula, if you don't stop, it's going to get a whole lot rougher for you," he blurted out in anger, shaking his finger at me.

"No . . . it can't get any rougher. Not after what you doctors have already put me through."

"Don't be bitter, Paula."

"I'll never be bitter, I won't give you doctors that victory. I call this the metamorphosis of Paula. I'm going to come out of this better than I have ever been before."

Forbes patted me on the cheek, and said, "I like the way you talk, Paula. You should go on TV."

"I'm thinking about it," I answered. "I need my breast cancer follow-up, and as that is not the part of me in litigation, can I have my scans and mammogram done here?"

"No, Paula! From now on you can only plan on having emergency treatment done here."

"Then you are telling me that I am forever blackballed in this town?"

"Yes, Paula."

"Okay, I'll go to Bay City Medical Center. That is a small price to pay for doing what I believe is right. But I want to leave this one thought with you: what would you do if what happened to me had happened to your wife or one of your daughters?"

It seemed as though he could finally relate to me as a real human being, because that question caused him to become teary eyed.

I continued, "The strangest thing of all is you're refusing to give me medical treatment, but I am the only one who is free to do what's right."

I was completely composed as I stood up, thanked him, and left his office.

As I was getting into my car, I suddenly heard the screeching of brakes. I turned and saw a very breathless Dr. Forbes running across the street. He had come within inches of getting run over by a passing car. He ran up the steps to the medical clinic where Dr. Post has his office. I had the feeling Dr. Forbes was reporting this latest "scoop" to Post.

I later learned that other people who have dared to sue our local doctors have also been denied medical treatment by our medical community. It seemed I had lots of company.

I admit I have never felt more utterly humiliated in all my life. My first reaction was to run and hide. I couldn't believe that the situation had deteriorated to such a degree. It was hard for me to believe that my only "crime" was that I had asked for the truth and that I was being punished.

My strong faith, again, carried me through.

That night, when I told Steve what had happened, he telephoned Forbes at his home and demanded an explanation. Forbes told Steve that he had been under peer pressure ever since he took me as a patient in October of 1978.

"Since that happened, Steve, my life has been miserable. None of the other doctors will even speak to me in the hospital halls. You just don't understand the system here in town. I had to dismiss Paula or else lose out on everything I've worked for all these years. All I'm trying to do is pay for a big house and raise my kids."

"You poor guy, you've really had it tough," Steve said in a fury. "While Paula's been having it so easy, here you've been suffering from terminal peer pressure. You really think that compares to the kind of hell she's been going through? Are we supposed to feel sorry for *you* now? Tell me, Forbes, when was the last time you guys gave a thought to your patient's welfare?"

"Look, Steve, I have to take orders like any other doctor in this town. If I don't, I stand to lose everything. Or maybe you don't know about the rigid indoctrination every new doctor faces when he first tries to set up practice here. He has to present himself at the head doctor's house—and I'm mentioning no names—and he is told how the medical profession is run in town. If he is willing to comply with all the rules and restrictions, he'll be permitted to succeed. If he isn't willing, he's told to take his act on the road. Of course, this is only implied, it's never an overt threat. If he absolutely refuses to be controlled and governed by the inner sanctum, it's made clear to him there's a bus leaving any minute. . . ."

"But who makes all these decisions?" Steve pressed him. "Who's putting all this pressure on you?"

"No more questions," Forbes said. "And if you repeat anything I've just told you, I'll deny everything and say you're lying." With that Forbes hung up.

I would later have cause to remember the special kind of peer pressure Forbes complained about when another woman sued a local doctor after he had maimed her daughter during a botched-up surgery. When that woman was badly injured a year later, she was refused medical treatment in town because she had dared to sue one of the doctors.

At the time, however, when Steve told me the gist of Forbes's conversation, I was newly appalled. Fortunately, all of the details of this conversation were well documented.

Chapter Fourteen

$\mathcal{T}$hat night, after my confrontation with Dr. Forbes, Steve and I went out to dinner. Who should be seated at the table next to us but Dr. and Mrs. Jud Kearny? Knowing what Forbes had told me that day, I felt certain that they were both amazed to see us out on the town, presumably celebrating. However, we had recognized their car in the parking lot as we drove up. When Steve asked if I wanted to go somewhere else, I said, "Don't be silly. I may be poison to every doctor here, but it's still a free country."

The way our tables were situated, Steve and Kearny sat back to back. Kearny and his wife seemed very tense and nervous, and I surmised it might be because Kearny had never dined that close to a victim before. But there were other friends of ours in the restaurant who stopped at our table to chat, while Steve and I carried on a light and joyful conversation.

As it happened, they left before we did. I greeted him with a bright smile. He said, "Good evening." Norma was extremely nervous and barely spoke.

The next day Steve called Flaky Floyd Lawrence at his office; he was still, more or less, serving as our attorney. Previously, we had told him to do nothing until he heard from us, so now he was hearing. Steve told him how Dr. Forbes had refused to treat me, and had advised me to go out of town for further medical service.

"Now that is really proof of a coverup," Lawrence said on the phone. "Let me take over now . . . and listen, I'm sorry for that misunderstanding before. As far as I'm concerned, I'm still your attorney of record, okay?"

What else could we do but agree at this late date? Lawrence said that if

91

Forbes had the gall to treat me like that, he was sure there had to be much more to the case than he had realized. As I had suspected, it was more than 'unethical' for Forbes to refuse to treat me.

During that same week in January, 1980, Steve also phoned his old friend, David Boylston, a retired dentist for whom I had once worked, a man who had certain connections with a few investigators working for MSB. Steve told him about the peer pressure being exerted against Forbes, adding, "Dave, I'll spend as much as one hundred thousand dollars to get to the bottom of this mess. I want proof as to who put Forbes up to handling Paula like this, who initiated the coverup, and exactly who it is Forbes has been taking orders from."

But Boylston, who was not an M.D. himself and hence, not a potential enemy, seemed genuinely unaware of what was going on in this case. And because he was definitely not a welcome member of the "in-group," it was understandable that they wouldn't include him in their private conspiracies.

At Steve's suggestion, Boylston telephoned an out-of-town investigator with the Medical Standards Board and said, "You'd better get up here fast—something big is happening."

On January 31st, I telephoned Dr. Nicholson in Bay City and told him what had been happening to me. He was shocked and truly sorry to hear what I had to tell him. "Paula, to me it's incredible that any reputable doctor would treat you this way. You are such a good patient, always so cooperative and uncomplaining." He was truly disturbed and upset for me; obviously he was mystified by this development, for I could tell it was news to him, and that he had not been in communication with Dr. Forbes. After I spoke with him, his receptionist made an appointment for me to see Nicholson on February 4th.

The next day Steve drove out of town to see Dr. Henderman, the first out-of-town doctor I had visited in March of 1978. He was also the doctor from whom Kearny had withheld certain records. Steve now showed Henderman all the records which Kearny had earlier refused to let him see.

Dr. Henderman studied these records, after which he sent letters to us verifying that he would have treated my case entirely differently had he been given access to all my records at the time he first saw me. He was not aware that Kearny had only performed a thyroid nodulectomy—a biopsy—until he read all the records. He further stated he would have done thyroid scans, thyroid panel blood tests, and so on. Like Nicholson, he too, was shocked by Kearny's behavior, and I still have his letter attesting to that.

Actually, Dr. Kearny had so craftily falsified the original records it led Dr.

Henderman to believe everything was fine. This was another part of Kearny's elaborate attempt to cover up his blunder during my thyroid surgery. The letter from Henderman utterly disputed the letter we had earlier received from our attorney's doctor-friend, his so-called "expert" witness who, for reasons still unknown, had said we had no case against Kearny.

On February 4th, I drove to Bay City to keep my appointment with Dr. Nicholson. He was still shocked and disturbed by the way the doctors had treated me.

"What puzzles me is that Dr. Forbes would give you an appointment when he knew he wasn't going to do the surgery for you. Certainly, that was unnecessarily cruel. He could have at least spared you the humiliation of going to his office by phoning you to discuss his intentions in advance. I just don't understand what's happening with those doctors. Someone in authority should have a talk with them."

This was the first time I had been shown genuine compassion from a doctor, and it touched me so deeply I couldn't hold back the tears. After Nicholson did his needle biopsy for me, I knew his gentle, sympathetic treatment of me had nothing to do with any phony bedside manner. Again I felt moved, telling myself that at last someone who is supposed to care really does care. At this time, that meant a great deal to me. Out of all the doctors I had seen who had manipulated me and lied to me, here was someone I could trust, someone who had real integrity and honor.

Of course, it was true that I had always been more agreeable and cooperative than any of those doctors deserved. In fact, the MSB investigator later assigned to our case once told me, "Paula, you did everything right. If you had been vehement or outraged, it would have been easy for them to write you off as a hysterical woman who wasn't responsible for her behavior, due to the severe nature of her illness."

Instead, I had continued to be quietly persistent, refusing to let the matter drop. I kept going back to confront these doctors, demanding answers. It would have been such a simple matter for four or five doctors to gang up on me and label me as having typically distraught or neurotic reactions to my ailment, or perhaps claim that these were side effects of my medication. They could well have said all of that, if I had lost control or behaved badly, and it would have been their expert word against mine, while they would come to the collective conclusion that I was acting under diminished capacity.

I sincerely believe they did everything in their power to get me to crack. They not only tried to sabotage my case with Lawrence, my attorney, they also pressured Dr. Forbes to drop me.

I'm glad to say I never behaved the way they expected me to. I kept my cool. Therefore, they could never imply that poor, suffering Mrs. Carroll had gone raving mad. It would also have been very easy for those doctors to spread the myth that all women who have had mastectomies go slightly off their rockers. The fact that I never once behaved as they had planned kept them confused and undecided as to how to handle me.

Late one night, two days after I had seen Dr. Nicholson, Steve got a surprise phone call from Dr. Post. When I heard Steve speak his name, I quickly picked up the extension phone and listened in on the conversation. We could tell at once that Dr. Post—the self-appointed "King" of the quacks—had been drinking heavily. He gave Steve the same ridiculous advice our attorney had given us earlier, saying we should sue Drs. Forbes and Nicholson. He also implied that he had "taken care of" our attorney. (Several months later when Post needed legal counsel to initiate a suit against his fellow doctors, he secured Lawrence to represent him.)

"I've been through Paula's records at the hospital," Post went on. Already he was confessing to something illegal, I thought, but knowing that Post's brother was the hospital administrator, it wasn't too difficult to figure out how he had gained access to my records. Yet he wasn't my doctor, so he had no right to see them. Also, by this time he had been served a ninety-day notice that he was going to be sued, so he was obviously getting panicky, going off-limits in more ways than one.

As it happened, Post's brother was one of only three people who had keys to those files, which meant the connection there was quite clear, though that didn't make it any less illegal.

During this conversation—which I had the presence of mind to completely document—Post also said, "I don't agree with what Dr. Nicholson is doing for Paula, Steve, so you'd better drop him. I wouldn't want to embarrass you in court; I don't want to make you look like a fool." It was ironic that Post would criticize the only responsible doctor who had ever treated me in this case. It almost looked as if he'd be much happier if I remained with the blunderers.

However, Post was really wound up that night. He did quite a monologue, most of it alcohol-induced, of course, though nonetheless revealing. "I've also been going over Paula's records at the pathology lab," he went on, "with the pathologist, Dr. Taylor. And by the way, I want to say I'm sorry for sending Paula that article, 'Doctor, Doctor, Cut My Throat.' It was a cowardly thing to do, to send it anonymously."

I knew the man had been drinking, but I still couldn't figure out how any man in his profession could allow himself to behave so sadistically towards a cancer patient. It was so cruel and careless as to be downright stupid, especially now, when in a loose moment, he was giving us this loquacious confession. Certainly he would never admit all this if he were sober, any more that he would voluntarily tell us he had gained illegal access to my medical records. He didn't know I was listening in on the extension, documenting every word he said, which made this a witnessed confession. I was still trying to figure out why they were fighting me so. It certainly wasn't to keep me from making a fool of myself. No, they were doing everything in their power to make me look like a fool, to discredit me, because they knew I knew the truth of what they did to me.

"You and Paula will make medical history if this ever gets to court," Post raved on, "because I'll make you both look like a couple of morons." Later during that same rambling conversation, the alcohol suddenly changed him from vitriolic to maudlin. Now he would have us believe he deeply cared what happened to me. "Listen, Steve, you and me, we go 'way back' so I'll tell you something: I spoke to a cancer specialist in Summerville." This told us he was still going safely far away from home for help. "His name is Dr. Steven Richards." It seemed even more weird that Post, who was not my doctor and, in fact, had refused to involve himself in my case two years earlier, was now discussing me with some doctor in Summerville. I wondered if his problems were due to drinking, or whether he had a dual personality; in either case, I was equally repelled.

During the last part of the phone conversation, Post insisted that I consult this cancer specialist in Summerville, though I felt sure he and his gang would be even happier if we moved there. Of course, any advice from Post—drunk or sober—would arouse my suspicions, as this definitely did. Steve and I had to wonder why our very worst enemy in this whole mess should suddenly express all this concern for us. It didn't make sense.

"Look, Doc," said Steve, "two years ago Paula begged you to take her case, and you practically kicked her out of your office. So why are you pretending you want to help her at this late date?"

"Good grief, fella, she was only five weeks post-op from her mastectomy at that time," said Post. "I couldn't touch her. You know that. It would have been unethical."

Hearing that, I recognized still another example of this man's warped values and priorities.

"While I've got you on the phone, Doc," Steve said, "I'd like to find out why you and Dr. Kearny pressured Forbes into dropping Paula?"

With that, Dr. Post actually managed to sound outraged. "Why that's not true. Where on earth did you hear such a lie?"

"From Dr. Forbes," said Steve. "Who else? And to hear him tell it, it was no lie. It was either drop Paula or he'd be dropped from the medical profession in town."

"Wait a minute, are you saying that Forbes accused me of pressuring him to drop Paula?"

"You talk to him about that," Steve hedged. From across the room I gave him a wink.

"Now look, Steve, I can't let this vicious gossip spread all over town. I have my reputation to uphold. How would it look to my patients if they knew I had to face a judge on questionable charges?"

"It would probably give them the first accurate impression they've ever had of you," Steve said pleasantly.

Post bypassed that and continued. "Damn it, you people can't do this to me. What're you trying to do, ruin my reputation? It's not fair!"

Steve had had quite enough. "After that idiotic remark, I think it's time you slept it off," he said, and together we hung up our phones.

That night Steve and I again wondered exactly how long it had been since any of those doctors had given a thought to my medical condition except, possibly, to wonder what was taking their "arch enemy" so long to expire. For months, every concern of theirs had involved nothing but petty politics and silly game playing. The fact that I had been seriously ill for some time no longer entered their minds.

Oddly enough, I had been so involved in all these conflicts and legal hassles, that I had been diverted from my illness to the point where I often lost sight of what I was fighting for. Or perhaps I had been replacing one agony for another. I was too determined to stop these doctors from ever hurting anyone else to ever sit back and wallow in self-pity or dwell exclusively on my medical symptoms. In that regard, our legal work was a positive activity, as it gave me so little time to concentrate on my condition. In any case, there was a limit to what *I* could do for myself medically; though I now felt there was a lot I could do to rectify the injustice done to me and spare others from the same treatment. For me, that was a true "reality incentive."

Not long after Post's call, my friend Penelope Beaumont, the wife of a local physician, called and said she had heard about Dr. Forbes refusing to treat me. "Paula," she said, "don't you dare let them scare you off. You're the only one who can stop what's going on with those doctors. Other people have tried but they have either been discredited or frightened off. Dr. Kearny must have that knife taken out of his hand. He has injured enough people. And to think, Paula, all he ever did on you was a biopsy . . . !"

"Why are they fighting me so?" I asked. "They have thrown everything but the kitchen sink at me."

Penelope answered, "Because these tricks have worked on others, and they didn't think you could live through the pressure after you found out the truth."

With that statement, she confirmed that all these doctors were determined to fight us with full artillery, hoping to intimidate us and finally scare us off. Yet I couldn't help remembering that before Dr. Forbes betrayed me, he did, literally save my life. For a time, this made him the one doctor in the group about whom I had mixed emotions.

On the other hand, it was Forbes's final cruelty toward me that lingered in my mind most emphatically, and I certainly couldn't condone the spineless way he deserted me when I needed him most. In the long run, that cancelled out all the good he had done for me prior to that episode. With his back against the wall, he chose corruption and deception. In my estimation, that's when he joined the ranks of the enemies.

He was now one of "them," more strongly dedicated to the cause of self-preservation than he was to the care of his patients.

He had sold out, and I was part of the price he had been willing to pay . . . .

Chapter Fifteen

On February 11, 1980, Steve and I felt we should play it safe and get a second opinion, just in case there was some basis of truth to Dr. Post's warning that we should get rid of Dr. Nicholson, though we both strongly doubted this. I still trusted Nicholson, no matter what Post had said about him on the phone. On the other hand, getting confirmation of Nicholson's diagnosis wouldn't hurt, so we consulted one of the best endocrinologists in the state, Dr. Arden.

Dr. Arden thoroughly examined me and reviewed all my medical records, and fully agreed with Dr. Nicholson that there had been serious mistakes, omissions, and coverups in the treatment of my thyroid cancer. He explained, "Dr. Kearny deliberately covered up his serious mistake, but he had to have had complete cooperation from the pathologists and the Tissue Committee. Your case involves criminal aspects because of the obvious conspiracy that existed between the doctors."

We were now satisfied that we had obtained an unbiased opinion. We also had expert confirmation of the fact that Kearny had committed many errors and omissions, but that Forbes and Nicholson had been correct in their diagnosis and treatment of me. Dr. Arden wrote a letter to me, documenting all the facts.

After we saw Dr. Arden, we also consulted with another attorney, a man who specialized in medical malpractice cases, though he usually served as a defense attorney for doctors. Although we hadn't officially dismissed our other attorney, he was still sitting dormant, doing no more active investigation for us, as Steve and I still didn't completely trust him. We couldn't forget his mistake with his consulting "doctor," and despite his denials, we still had an idea he was in direct contact with

Dr. Post. However, we dared not dismiss him until we had another attorney who was willing to handle our case.

This attorney, whose name was Stillman, definitely believed we had a case. However, he warned me that the damages I could prove would be minimal, because I was still alive (where had I heard that before?). But now that we had proof of the deliberate coverup, those amounted to punitive damages, which malpractice insurance does not cover.

Stillman also pointed out that most of my complaint was criminal because of the blatant conspiracy that existed between Kearny, the hospital's Tissue Committee, and the pathologists. He further pointed out that the Mayo Clinic letters proved all this. Stillman advised me to contact the local district attorney and MSB. He further stated, "With those Mayo Clinic letters, you can never be discredited. They prove your civil and criminal case."

Believing, of course, that we definitely had a case, Stillman put us in touch with a prestigious law firm in Bay City—Sorrenson and Galton. They specialized in medical malpractice cases for the patient, not the doctors. After reviewing our case, these people agreed to handle it. Vincent Galton, one of the partners, offered to handle my case personally, so it was he who actually filed the court action against Kearny and Post.

Now we felt secure enough to cancel our contract with "Flaky" Lawrence. When we contacted him, he said, "Paula, I'd really like to continue with your case. It's one of the most unusual cases I have ever seen, and it intrigues me." He rambled on about how he was his own man and never yielded to pressure from anyone.

"But I suppose I have damaged my credibility with you," he added.

"Damaged it?" I said. "You've scuttled it completely. I couldn't trust you in a court, as you were so quick to dump me before." Thankfully, we had found Vincent Galton before the statute of limitations ran out, so that officially ended my relationship with Floyd Lawrence.

As it happened, on March 3rd, Mr. Galton filed our case just six hours before the statute of limitations ran out, right under the wire. Those were frantic weeks for us, with Steve running one way and me running another in our effort to get everything together on time. There was a whole month of furious and involved activity. At times it all seemed so wildly incredible.

About this time Steve got in touch with an old friend of his who had recently retired from the FBI after twenty-five years of service as an agent. As he now had his own private investigator's license, Steve asked Fred if he would do a little investigating for us. He agreed.

Steve told him something I had found out earlier.

"Fred, I've heard that Forbes's wife Thelma has publicly made the statement that the reason Forbes left the offices of Drs. Robins and Kearny was because those two were 'a couple of butchers.' "

"Okay," said Fred. "I'll go out and interview Mrs. Forbes and see why she made such a statement." He added that if he got further information from this talkative lady, it might be something our attorney could use in our case.

Of course, everybody in town knew that Thelma Forbes was a compulsive gossip. She had been making these damaging statements in front of witnesses, knowing they could harm her husband.

Anyway, our good friend Fred Augustine, the investigator, went to Thelma Forbes's house and asked her point-blank: "I've been told you have been telling everyone that your husband describes Drs. Kearny and Robins as the 'town butchers.' Is that correct?"

This took her so unawares, she could do nothing but stammer and splutter for a few seconds. Finally, she uttered a few innocuous words. "Well, I can't comment. That is privileged information." She refused to answer any of his further questions. She should have simply denied his first implication, because her failure to deny implied an admission.

When Dr. Forbes got home that night, his rattled wife must have told him that Fred had grilled and interrogated her to the point of hysteria. Or else, Forbes got hysterical himself when he realized exactly what oft-repeated rumor Fred had questioned her about. Whatever the reason, Dr. Forbes called Fred's home that night, and Fred later reported that the man sounded like he was totally out of his mind; Fred had found it difficult to remember he was talking to a professional man.

"You know, Paula," Fred said when describing this frantic phone conversation, "I've interrogated communists, Mafia members, even psychos, but I've never known a man to go so totally off the wall on the telephone. Let's hope he wasn't scheduled for surgery the next day. I'll tell you something else: judging by the way this guy overreacted, I'd say your case is just the tip of the iceberg. These doctors must have been covering up an awful lot of blunders which no other patient called them on, or blew the whistle the way you're doing. Imagine what they must have been getting away with all these years, and how many terminal cases they've created by their substandard treatment."

Around this time, in late February of 1980, Mr. Kenyon, an investigator with MSB, came to town to consult with me, at which time I presented my case to him. He, too, branded it "blackmail and conspiracy." When he read of how Post had given me seventy-two Dalmane capsules without entering it it in his records, he said, "They gave you a loaded gun and hoped you would use it." Of course, I had already suspected this earlier.

Kenyon complimented me for being the only person from our town to ever stand up to a local doctor. He said, "The people in this town are a bunch of chickens. They are afraid to stand up to the bad medicine that is practiced here; it is some of the worst in the state. I guess, in a way, they deserve what they get. Let me tell you this: don't ever go into one of their hospitals; the doctors would make a mistake for sure. Everyone is entitled to make a mistake and they'd make one for sure in your case."

When Kenyon went to the hospital to pick up my records, he observed at once that the clerk had withheld some of the documents. How he knew those records were missing, I'm not sure, though I assume it was part of his agency's overall investigation.

Kenyon demanded the rest of the records, whereupon he and the clerk got into an argument. Fortunately, at that very moment the Accreditation Team was conducting a routine inspection of the hospital. The doctor in charge of this team overheard the commotion with Kenyon and the clerk and got involved in their quarrel. As he knew Kenyon personally, the doctor went up and said, "What's the trouble, Howard?"

"Would you believe it, Paul," said Kenyon, "these people tried to short-sheet me some records. Maybe if you tell them who they're dealing with, they'll get on the ball."

The accreditation doctor eyed the clerk and shook his head in dismay. "Shame on you," he said. "You give this man all the records he needs. If he's conducting an investigation for the state, you are required by law to give him whatever he's asking for." It was then that the clerk went to the files and found that all my records were missing. Later the hospital was written up for this attempt to withhold evidence, which the Accreditation Team viewed as a serious infraction.

Upon being told the records were "temporarily" missing, Kenyon told the clerk he would sit right there until those documents showed up.

This was on a Wednesday, which happened to be Dr. Post's day off. It was common knowledge that Post usually got drunk at home every Wednesday. However, in this emergency the clerks phoned him at home, telling him to get down to the hospital at once to help them search for the missing records.

Post didn't have to stagger far to find those missing records. They were in his office at the clinic where he worked. They had been brought there by his brother, the hospital administrator. Not only was it illegal for these records to be in Post's possession; he was also guilty of downright thievery: removing confidential records from the hospital to his personal office. We now had irrefutable proof that Dr. Post had gained illegal access to my personal medical records.

During that same visit, Mr. Kenyon provided me with some other "interesting" insights as to what the local doctors were up to.

"Don't worry, Mrs. Carroll," he said, "the state knows what's happening here. A couple of years ago I asked your district attorney to issue warrants for three local doctors, but he refused. So I had to call the state attorney general's office to get those warrants, one of which involved a morals offense. That action authorized me to make arrests, which is exactly what I did."

"You arrested three local doctors?" I asked, astonished.

"I sure did," Kenyon replied. "That's why the town's doctors still have it in for me. Not long after those arrests, I met with some of your local doctors in an attempt to help them avoid patient complaints. But they gave me such a bad time, interrupting me every time I opened my mouth, I couldn't present my program. After the meeting, one of the doctors followed me out to my car and said, "Mr. Kenyon, you have no idea what's going on here." So I said, "Okay, fill me in." And he proceeded to enlighten me about a lot of shocking truths, the details of which I won't go into now, except to tell you they're worse than anything you've suspected."

Before he left, Kenyon cornered several of the hospital's chief administrators and said, "You tell these doctors to stop their intimidation of Paula Carroll, as their actions are illegal."

Meanwhile, during the same day, after Kenyon left the hospital, the doctors called a special meeting. During that meeting—and we now have proof of this, also—the doctors put Dr. Kearny through a grinding inquisition, keeping him on the hot seat for four hours.

At this time many of our loyal friends let us know how they admired us for having the courage not to give up our battle against the local medical incompetents. They also admired the fact that we had never once considered closing up our business or leaving town. Steve and I knew that was never even a serious consideration for us. This was our home, and our business was something we had worked hard to build up together. So we were staying put.

The support of our loyal friends meant a great deal to us at this time. Yet we still had to contend with Dr. Kearny's loyal supporters, those misguided souls who still believed this man was everything he appeared to be. I had to wonder how many of these "friends" had also been patients of this man. I still kept getting phone calls from people who bitterly condemned me for vilifying this honorable man and threatening his reputation. This continued to be my most difficult struggle, having to face the public scorn of people who firmly believed Dr. Kearny was a gentle, civic-minded citizen, a man of true integrity. In their eyes, I remained the guilty one. They had become so used to the practice of bad medicine that they no longer realized what constituted good medicine. Some of the "insiders" had compromised their values and justified bad results with little more than a shrug.

It was also very heartwarming for me when several medical personnel—nurses, doctors, and others—let me know they were one hundred percent *for* what I was doing, telling me how they approved my attempt to fight the system. This confirmed what I had already known, that not every doctor and nurse in town swore allegiance to Dr. Kearny and his group and their substandard medicine.

It was good to know that some members of our medical community wanted something done to change the gross inequities that had been tolerated and covered up for so many years. They felt this kind of fight had to be waged by an outsider, not by one of them.

Yet I feel there's another way to look at this situation: in time these professionals are the people who *must* report on their malpracticing colleagues, for surely, in the final analysis, effective change can only be brought about from within the system. Unfortunately, we're again up against the unwritten law here: it's so rare that one doctor will testify against another, no matter how bitterly, or privately, because he is unwilling to condemn the other's procedures or policies. Most doctors feel that anything that makes "the professional" look bad should be kept quiet. So the honest ones stand by and watch, hoping that some wronged patient will take action to stop the medical misfits among them. This can be a terribly long wait, particularly when the aforementioned wronged patient doesn't even know or suspect the wrong that has been committed against him.

It is my fervent hope that in time members of the medical profession will evolve some discreet, albeit effective, method to police and monitor one another. Perhaps there could be a simple method established whereby they could turn in a blundering colleague anonymously, without ever having it revealed who it was that pointed the finger.

In view of the anachronistic tradition of silence and secrecy among doctors and nurses, one wonders how many other autonomous medical dictatorships might be flourishing in small, isolated towns throughout the country, and how many other hushed-up surgical crimes are being tolerated?

As for what had been going on in the community itself, I eventually learned how unprecedented my action was. Until I tiptoed onto the scene, very few patients had ever dared to sue a local doctor.

Chapter Sixteen

*D*uring the early spring of 1980, when I realized I was officially without a doctor in town, I took Dr. Nicholson's advice and found a doctor closer to me than he was. I had heard that my childhood doctor had recently moved his practice about forty miles out of town. Dr. George Middleton knew me from giving me yearly checkups in the past, though he had no idea about my case.

I asked Middleton to take over my case and work with Dr. Nicholson. I gave him a brief rundown on my recent medical history, then told him in great detail exactly what had happened and why I couldn't get treatment locally. When I told him my story I was, at first, very apprehensive as to how he would react, wondering if I faced still another medical rejection. Once again I was in the absurd position of having to beg a doctor to treat me, two and a half years after my first cancer surgery. It seemed so ludicrous and degrading.

Middleton listened carefully to my story. Then he said, "Paula, even if I didn't know you or know where you were from, after hearing your story I'd have no doubt what town you were talking about. After what I've personally witnessed there, nothing about those doctors could ever surprise me again. This sort of thing has been going on there for years, though I'm grateful I managed to stay clear of it. I know for a fact that some of the surgeons often go into the operating room drunk, and they're constantly bickering among themselves. I could tell you horror stories about those doctors that might even surprise *you*. That's why I believe every word you're telling me."

In any case, Middleton wanted me to know he didn't feel in the least threatened by my litigation, and he assured me he would be happy to work with Dr. Nicholson on my case.

I spoke to Middleton for about forty-five minutes that day, and when I was about to leave, he asked me if he had spent enough time with me. I told him, "You've spent more time with me in one visit than any one of my home town doctors have spent with me collectively over the last two and a half years." I further assured him that his willingness to listen to me had been so rare that it was therapeutic. He had no ax to grind, so he was one of the doctors I could talk to without worrying about his hidden or ulterior motives.

Perhaps I should have gone to him first; perhaps if he had still been practicing in town at the time, I might have. But in the beginning, if you'll recall, I wanted someone "familiar" and close to home. Besides, there were already too many "should-haves" in my case.

I had been told by Dr. Nicholson that I would only need a general practitioner at this time, which was why he advised me against returning to Dr. Henderman, who also practiced in the same nearby town as Dr. Middleton. Henderman was a specialist who offered the same kind of treatment that Nicholson still meant to provide for me at Bay City Medical Center. Hence, my choice of Dr. Middleton.

Just to know that Middleton was genuinely concerned for me, and to realize I had a specialist like Nicholson in my corner, made me feel secure about my medical future for the very first time. This proved to me there were caring doctors after all and that, hopefully, the medical corruption that flourished in some areas was, at least relatively speaking, an exception to the rule. I just happened to be in the wrong town at the wrong time. After all, some members of the local medical profession wanted this corruption stopped.

It is vitally important for the patient to realize that not all medicine is equal in quality and not all doctors are equal in their abilities to practice medicine.

Recently, while I was up at Bay City Medical Center, as I was waiting to see the chief surgeon, I overheard members of the staff talking with a woman who was about to have a mastectomy the next morning. She'd already had a biopsy, and it had proved malignant. I was both impressed and amazed to hear how thoroughly all her questions were answered by the staff. These people told her exactly what to expect, counseled her in advance for a full half hour, and gave her the sort of medical enlightenment nobody ever thought to give me when I faced the same kind of surgery at the hands of Dr. Kearny.

Now, after what seemed like centuries later, I was finding out what I had missed. It was so rewarding to know this kind of advance counseling was being offered in other hospitals, and that the frightened patient was not left in total ignorance as to what she could expect.

When I overheard all that, I felt like a remnant from the Dark Ages. Now I saw the light, gratified to know it wasn't too late for others to be handled correctly by such professionals.

Chapter Seventeen

*I*t is interesting—albeit disheartening—to discover what a near-impossible task a person takes on when he decides to sue for malpractice. The system puts up such a fight when a private citizen attempts such a suit that one attorney told us he wouldn't consider a malpractice case unless he was guaranteed a minimum fee of fifty thousand dollars. That's because it takes an attorney four times as much time and work to prepare a malpractice case as it does other civil suits.

The medical profession spends millions of dollars to protect itself against malpractice suits. Thus, it is all but impossible for a patient to take legal action against a guilty doctor even when such action is justified. Unfortunately, the medical profession continues to ignore the real truth, which is that malpractice suits can only be restrained by a more humane concern for the patient. This could be done by stopping the consistently negligent physicians and hospitals.

It is estimated that only one case in ten incidents of malpractice result in a claim, and less than half of these, one in twenty-five, receive payment.[1]

This fact is contrary to all the press releases issued through the medical profession's public relations firms. One county medical association recently proposed to assess each physician in the county one thousand dollars a year for an advertising campaign extolling the virtues of organized medicine. It seems as if the medical profession has never heard that a healthy, satisfied customer is the best advertisement.

In fact, in 1976, thanks to an unwitting social experiment in Los Angeles, we were given proof of how much healthier the public would be if they stayed away from doctors and hospitals. If you'll recall, due to the fast-rising cost of medical malpractice insurance, there was a doctors' strike in Los Angeles that year. It lasted for thirty-five days. What happened during that period was no coincidence: the death rate went way down. The longer the strike lasted, the fewer people died.[2]

It is futile for a patient who has been medically wronged to register a legal complaint. The expertise with which medical incompetence is hidden and unpunished by the secretive medical fraternity, and the law itself, is testimony to this sad fact. This conspiracy of silence is all part of an expert defense system established over the years by medicine against its natural enemy—the injured, dissatisfied patient.

In some cases, the injured patient is brainwashed into believing that the malpractice was their fault for failing to understand how the system works. Some critics firmly believe that the patient should remain silent even when there is a legitimate malpractice claim. Their myopic reasoning is that malpractice is caused by the patient, not the physician or hospital. They would rather stifle the patient's right to challenge another than challenge the negligence that gave rise to the claim.

A physician recently explained to a patient and family: "Hospitals are there for your use—use them at your own risk." With this sort of attitude, it would seem appropriate that we place warning signs on the front doors of these institutions: THE SURGEON-GENERAL HAS DETERMINED THAT THIS FACILITY COULD BE HAZARDOUS TO YOUR HEALTH.

There is a blatant refusal by medicine and government to police doctors who are guilty of gross negligence. This indicates the laxity of both the profession and our existing laws. The AMA has said that all too seldom are licensed physicians called to task by boards, societies, or colleagues. It is the tendency of such groups to shield, rather than censure, offending colleagues. Physicians can even continue unchecked by our medical disciplinary system, the Medical Standards Board. In 1982, 5,000 complaints were filed with the MSB and 175 disciplinary actions were taken. The MSB points to their record with pride, claiming it's the best in the country. I suppose that is like proclaiming, "We're the best of the worst."

It is always humorous to hear how quickly the critics of malpractice change their minds when it is they or their loved ones who are harmed by inferior medical care. As long as malpractice happens to someone else, they exude a smugness and self-righteous air against anyone who would dare to sue a hospital or doctor. They must reason: a malpractice law suit is never justified *except* when it happens to me or my family.

One such person, who recently underwent surgery, refused to sign the arbitration agreement that would have limited his rights to sue if he became a victim of malpractice during his surgery and hospitalization. The doctor asked him why, and he answered, "I am the sole supporter of my family and if anything happens to me, I've told them to sue the socks off of you."

I recently attended a Society of Law and Medicine conference where Patricia Danzon, an economist at Duke University, reported from her studies: "The allegation that malpractice insurance is a major factor driving the high and rising cost of health care is exaggerated. Between 1975 and 1982 malpractice premiums rose roughly seventy-three percent, while the cost of a physician's services rose ninety-two percent, and the cost of a hospital room rose 130 percent. Overall, malpractice insurance premiums account for around one percent of the total 350 billion dollar health care bill. For physicians, malpractice insurance premiums average around three percent of their annual gross income, which is currently estimated at around 200 thousand dollars."

Patricia Danzon continues, "Why are medical providers and other professionals exposed to tort liability for professional negligence, while most other occupations are still exempt? The answer lies in the information gap between professionals and their clients. If the patient were as knowledgeable as the physician about the cost, benefits, and risks of alternative treatments and the quality of care being received, the patient could protect his own interests."

Mrs. Danzon pointed out that the full social cost of injuries due to malpractice is probably several times greater than the more visible costs of malpractice claims.

A study made by the U.S. Census Bureau indicates that the average malpractice premium per physician actually declined by 6.5 percent from 1977 to 1981. It was shown that even neurosurgeons, who pay the highest percentage of gross income of any specialty, spend only 5.8 percent. Fifty-seven percent of doctors spend less than five thousand dollars on malpractice premiums and only twelve percent spend over fifteen thousand dollars.[3]

Richard Shandell, a New York trial lawyer, said New York City doctors pay the highest premiums in the country, yet they pay a smaller percentage of their gross income on liability insurance than does a New York cab driver.[4]

In a recent medical malpractice lawsuit, the defendant physician who had chosen to "go bare" (i.e., he did not have any malpractice insurance), nonchalantly announced, "If the jury gives me a guilty verdict, I'll file bankruptcy. They (the injured patient) won't get a dime from me."

111

This particular lawsuit was the seventh malpractice claim that has been filed against this physician. He is a bitter man, without remorse for the needless human suffering his incompetence and greed have caused. Furthermore, and most disturbing, he feels no responsibility to his victims.

It is a well-known fact that the medical lobbyists are all-powerful at the state and federal levels. Their influence over the way our elected officials vote on health care issues is testimony to their biases that favor not the consumer but the "medical-industrial complex." The enormous financial contributions that elected officials receive sway many a vote in favor of the system.

An MSB official recently lamented, "Whenever we challenge a doctor for self-abuse of drugs or incompetency we can always expect a call from his elected representative telling us what a fine man this doc is and how any disciplinary action would ruin his exemplary reputation." No one ever asks, "What about the poor patient?" It is always, "What about the poor doctor?" How many people must suffer before we put the question in its proper perspective?

A short time ago I talked with one of the state's leading medical malpractice attorneys. He explained that one case took him two years to prepare and cost ninety thousand dollars of his own money. The doctor had failed to diagnose breast cancer in a twenty-eight-year-old woman. This doctor's negligence lead to her untimely death; she left behind a grieving husband and two small children. Testimony showed that the doctor failed to provide the acceptable standard of care and that her chances of complete cure were excellent had she been correctly diagnosed when she was first examined. The jury refused to rule against the doctor because he was a "pillar of the community."

The jury's verdict did not alter the fact that this "grandfatherly" doctor's negligence caused a needless death. Although the jury did not find in favor of the plaintiff's survivors, this did not mean the doctor was innocent of wrongdoing, it just meant that his insurance didn't have to pay for it.

No one case, no matter how horrible and significant it might be, will accomplish the needed reforms. I caution people who are considering the possibility of filing a malpractice suit to first consider all of the energy they will expend and the disappointments they will experience when they launch upon this endeavor. The heartbreak that these innocent victims must endure is beyond the average person's comprehension.

The more I see others and witness their experiences with the malpractice system, the more I become convinced that we must look for ways to prevent malpractice from happening in the first place. Human error is understandable, but how much is permissible when it is repeated over and over again?

Everyone knows the real victim is the patient, but there is another group of victims whose suffering is less well known. These real victims are the ones who actually pay for the increased insurance premiums because of physician and hospital negligence. These are the people that suffer physical and emotional damage and even death in some cases.

A word of caution is in order to those within the medical profession who so freely criticize attorneys for causing the malpractice crisis. Without the legal counsel of some of the most expensive attorneys, these very doctors would be in jail for medical welfare fraud and drug abuse, or for other illegal acts. According to one of the MSB's investigators, "If we (the general public) do something considered to be illegal, we end up going to jail . . . . These doctors never go to jail . . . very rarely ever."

The injured patients are thrown into circumstances beyond their control and there is virtually no recourse for them. The victimized patient always starts on his quest for justice from a position of absolute weakness. He may have permanent disabilities because of the doctor's negligence, so his capabilities of facing a challenge are minimized. Also, he may be unfortunate enough to have a less than caring or competent attorney in his corner. On the other side...there is an attorney for each doctor named in the suit, the hospital's attorneys, plus all of the insurance companies' attorneys and powerful investigators. Uneven odds? The deck is stacked against you before you even start. If your case is so blatant that there is no way anyone from the defense can confuse the issues with clever talk, you are in for some sobering surprises. Then, and only then, do you understand who the *real* victims are.

Can you imagine anyone choosing to put themselves through such an experience because, as their detractors would have us believe, they are litigious or they want to "make a lot of money?" There is not one of the hundreds of people I know that were forced into these conditions that wouldn't gladly reverse the effects of the circumstances that gave rise to the filing of a claim.

Aggrieved doctors, or hospitals, never hesitate to seek justice through a court of law if they, or their families or possessions, have been damaged. Because of their financial position and prestige they can buy the best attorney to represent them.

One of the most ridiculous cases involved a doctor's family, who sued a contractor for breaking a fireplace brick in their home with damages estimated at eighty dollars. Yet, anytime this physician has been sued for his repeated incompetence a loud protest goes up from his friends and supporters condemning the offending person for filing a lawsuit against "such a fine man."

What gave rise to this double standard? Is it to be understood that the only one that is to be excused with the comment "it was an honest human error" is the doctor? Why should this be, when his repeated negligent acts have caused much more suffering than did a broken brick? Should they be the only ones allowed, because of their elevated positions, to seek and be granted legal remedies? Why aren't they able to admit they are not perfect, admit their mistakes, and *learn* from them? This revelation may be a surprise to some within the medical community, but the average person no longer views the doctor as "godlike."

It would seem that for many doctors, medical ethics consists of never revealing the truth to the patient. As one physician states, when faced with glaring evidence of another doctor's mistake, medical ethics dictate that only the doctor who made the mistake is informed of it, never the patient. This so-called "ethical method" also includes not even raising one's eyebrows when faced with the evidence of another doctor's mistake. To sum it up, medical ethics, to some, means not getting caught.

I have personally experienced this kind of performance: the charade wherein doctors pretend they don't notice any irregularity at all, even though they know on sight that something is drastically wrong.

During my visits with many cancer patients, I couldn't fail to notice how negligently and callously many of these terminally ill patients were treated by the hospital staff. Of course, remembering my own experiences, it came as no surprise to me that a kind of instant war is declared whenever an unsuspecting patient is admitted to a hospital. It is always "them" against you. And because your enemy is well and healthy and armed to the teeth—with pills and surgical tools—and you are sick and defenseless, there is really no contest. Your only choice is to surrender without even putting up a fight.

The more I thought about that situation, the more angry I became. I asked myself: if these people can't defend themselves, why can't the rest of us step in and at least *try* to fight their battles for them? How else can we balance the scales of justice unless we average citizens band together and rise up in protest?

Little did I know at the time exactly how far that question would take me, or in which direction. Are you ready for a mild-mannered Paula Carroll in the role of flaming activist? Neither was I!

[1] Goddard, Thomas G., "The American Medical Association is Wrong—There is no Medical Malpractice Insurance Crisis," *The Los Angeles Daily Journal-Report* 85-10:17.

[2] In one Los Angeles tabloid the headlines blared: *"Doctors Go On Strike—Death Takes A Holiday!"*

[3] Statistical Abstract of the US, 1984, Bureau of Census, US Department of Commerce, p.111, and AM Best's Casualty Loss Reserve Development, 1978, through 1984.

[4] Ibid, pp. 16-17.

Chapter Eighteen

*I*t all began to happen for me when, in the spring, of 1981, I gave
a series of interviews to a news reporter by the name of Nick
Andrews. He had already done some investigative reporting on the cases
of rampant medical abuse in our area, and was also familiar with the harrowing experiences I had encountered on my own. I met with him a
number of times that spring and summer and he soon became a very supportive confidante for me.

One day he told me he had all the information he needed for his report,
but added, ". . . except for the big finish. That's where you come in,
Paula. You're the only one who can give this material the dramatic punch
it needs to get the right attention."

"Me, dramatic?" I laughed, certain he was kidding. "I'm about as
dramatic as Little Bo Peep, only taller."

"That's why you'd make such an ideal leader, if you started your own
consumer advocate group," he said. "I mean, the doctors here are going
crazy with all the power they've been given. Isn't it time you did something more positive than simply consoling the battered?"

I looked at him. "Oh, Nick, you must have been reading my mind.
I've been thinking of doing something like that for months, but I guess I
was waiting for someone more . . . well, more powerful to step in and do
it for me."

"No, you wouldn't want to do this sort of thing with too much power, not
in that stifled little town. You don't want to scare them. You want to educate
them. And you have just the right kind of "soft-sell" approach to make it
work. Believe me, you'll get a lot more messages across if you come on like
the lady you are, instead of some shrill and militant feminist."

"You know, Nick, for some funny reason, that almost makes sense to me," I said. "It's as if the more softly I speak, the more attention people will have to pay in order to hear what I'm saying."

"Exactly!" he said. "But if you were a screamer, all they'd hear would be the anger of your tone, and they would completely disregard the content of what you're saying."

"Hmm," I murmured reflectively, " 'speak softly but carry a big stick. . .' "

"Right, and your 'big stick' would be facts and documentation and research. You'd be armed with knowledge and the kind of information that would prevent others from becoming the sort of near-fatal victim you almost were."

That brief discussion was the beginning of a very big change in my life and as it turned out, in the lives of so many others who, until our group got going, were convinced they were at the end of their rope. After that talk with Nick, I went home and did some in-depth studying at the local Law Library, where the area's professional lawyers and law students do their research. I boned up on the legal aspects of setting up my own consumer advocate group. I thoroughly researched the medical-legal field, learning how to draw up my own incorporation papers, and file for and obtain both my federal and state tax exemptions.

Because of my naiveté, or my beginner's luck, I didn't realize how difficult it would be to get such exemptions. Now I'm glad I didn't, as I would probably have hesitated and thought it over. This way, not knowing how "impossible" it was, I plunged right ahead. I sent off letters for both my state and federal tax exemptions, explaining my intention to organize a free medical service geared to the public, and I was granted both exemptions without hesitation.

That meant that all public donations sent to our group, as well as my business expenses, would be tax-deductible. And because of this tax-exempt status, I've also become eligible for all the surplus material and equipment provided by the state, which I will need if, and when, I set up a private center outside of my home. By the time I'm able to finance this move, I'll have access to typewriters, computers, desks—all of which are government surplus merchandise I can purchase for a pittance, as long as I only use this equipment for my consumer group.

But all that would come later. At the start, it took quite a bit of doing to get this project off the ground. But thanks to the publicity generated by Nick Andrews when his articles were published nationwide, plus some well-timed TV exposure, Paula Carroll's new movement was soon being talked about all over the state. Officially, we call ourselves Consumers

For Medical Quality, Inc., and the main focus of our organization is to help people get through the health care system.

It was easy for me to identify with some of the problems other frightened patients experience, because in the beginning, I, too, was naive, unschooled, trusting, and unquestioning, not to mention intimidated by the pompous mystique of the medical profession; and, let's face it, I was downright dumb! Except for getting that second opinion in time to save my life, I did everything wrong. Now, perhaps, others could profit by my early failures and learn, as I had via the simple means of self-enlightenment, how to turn those failures into successes.

Officially, our group got going in September of 1981, with Steve as our instant, though not always silent, partner whenever he could spare the time from his business. Only one month later, thanks mostly to Nick Andrews's articles, we had already received more than 175 letters and hundreds of telephone inquiries from far and wide. The letters came from as far away as Illinois and Missouri, presumably from people who had read the news articles.

Meanwhile, Steve and I converted one of our guest bedrooms into the library. I had already amassed a great number of reference books while doing my own medical research which, if you'll remember, was a process that helped to save my life.

However, once the word was out, I had a feeling we'd get a lot more books as donations. So Steve and I proceeded to line all the walls with shelves. He initially felt that would be overdoing it a bit, but later that same week, when a nearby hospital donated over 200 medical books to our library, he had to admit those extra shelves would come in handy.

Eventually, we had as many as 500 medical volumes in our home-library, which is one of the largest medical libraries of its kind ever owned by a layperson. We also have thousands of brochures and pamphlets and, in time, we were given computer access to the National Institutes of Health in Bethesda, Maryland.

Among my many goals, I planned to make available to the layman the kind of information that was previously accessible only to the medical professional. Usually, when average patients ask their doctors vital questions about their condition, they are placated, humored, and in general, treated as if they are children. In fact, doctors will often say anything to *avoid* giving their patient an intelligent answer. I believe that some doctors don't even know the answers and then try to hide behind the feeble excuse that the " . . . patient won't understand."

As I've said on several TV talk shows and in many newspaper interviews, "I feel it's time for us to ask why, and in this way help to demythologize this exalted and ridiculously deified profession. Usually, by the time most people go to their doctors, they're too sick to fight back when their kindly physician starts to manipulate them. Now they have a place to go when they're in doubt.''

It was amazing how quickly the people who needed us found out about our group. It appeared, right from the start, that we had found a need and we were filling it. We began getting calls and written inquiries from as many as twenty-two states. In no time at all, our group began to receive more calls than the local referral service.

Our service is free of charge and financed entirely by private contributions. It is strictly an information service—I don't attempt to treat or diagnose any of the people who appeal to us for help. Mostly, I familiarize them with their rights. If they ask, I give them the latest research on some particular ailment. For example, they might want to know the newest treatment for asthma, or the latest advances being made in the field of nutrition and vitamins. I do the research for them in my library, then I photocopy the resulting material and mail it to them. I might also deliver it in person. I've met some of the nicest people that way. In time, however, I also had many willing volunteers who helped me write letters and take care of the many other clerical duties that began to pile up.

We were soon inundated by donated research materials from the medical libraries of a number of respected universities and medical centers throughout the United States. Within a very few months, we started publishing our quarterly ''Monarch Newsletter.'' The name evolved from our corporate logo, which is based on the monarch butterfly. To me, this is the symbol of regeneration and new life. This publication deals with patients' rights to know about such things as mastectomies, hysterectomies, and Caesarean sections; how to find advocates and specialists for second opinions; and where to call for taped informational messages. In time, some of our longer essays began to tackle such themes as ''Making Decisions Under Stress.''

Looking back, it seems astonishing to think how quickly we were launched by our own momentum, and how, once we knew exactly what we were doing, we were determined to keep on doing it. Much to my personal delight, during my extensive research I found that a great deal of this material fascinated me in ways I had never expected. Due to this serendipity, I immensely enjoyed this invaluable fringe benefit. Not only was I learning what I would need to know to head up this group, but I was genuinely engrossed by the process. In short, I was turning myself into an accomplished research technician and having a whale of a time just doing my homework.

Only a few weeks after our group got underway, I received a call from a local family who told me a story of such appalling medical abuse, it provided the final motivation I needed to convince me how desperately the public needed our services.

This case involved the two sons of an elderly hospital patient who, they claimed, had died from criminal neglect and abuse. When the sons saw that their seventy-four-year-old father was being mistreated to the point where he was literally left to die of neglect, they tried to get him released from the hospital. But the hospital authorities refused to permit this and threatened to have the sons arrested if they attempted to take their father out of the hospital on their own. Indeed, when one of the sons tried this, they called the police and had him handcuffed.

Initially, the old man was admitted to the hospital due to a minor stroke and other ailments related to aging, though none of these ailments were life-threatening at the time of his admission. A few months later he was dead as a result of the many complicating ailments he contracted while he was a patient. In short, as his sons maintained, it was the treatment, or the lack of treatment, he received in that hospital that finally killed him. Only a few days before his death, the old man suffered a stroke and was left unattended for two hours on a gurney in one of the hospital's deserted hallways.

After his death, the coroner notified the police, as it appeared to him that the deceased had been murdered, judging by the amount of bruises on his body, plus the visible signs of abuse and long neglect. The poor man weighed only fifty pounds when he died. The autopsy listed the causes of death as cardiac arrhythmia with severe arteriosclerosis, mild pneumonia, liver congestion, and ulcerated bedsores. The man had had none of these deteriorating ailments when he was admitted.

When I spoke to the two sons, they told me he was literally starved and beaten to death. They had taken photographs of the corpse which were suggestive of victims in Nazi concentration camps. When they told me of their futile attempt to have the case investigated by MSB, I had a touch of *deja vu*, recalling the many brick walls I had run up against in seeking justice. They went to various lawyers, wrote a senator, the FBI. But they were repeatedly told that their proper course of action lay with local authorities—the same authorities, the family believed, who had failed to follow up on the investigation in the first place.

I spoke to Nick Andrews, and together we were able to generate some publicity about this case. The shocking story was told in a number of newspapers throughout the state.

The grief and frustration encountered by that one family convinced me of the vicious catch-22-type futility average citizens experience whenever they try to follow up their suspicions of medical authorities.

This family needed help from a group with no ax to grind, and, as it turned out, our corporation became one of the few organizations in town that could make that statement. As a nonprofit agency, we were in business to serve an embattled public, not to feed on their misfortunes. From the very beginning, we made that clear to the people who needed us.

Many of the following case-histories are composite, though well-documented, stories of some of the horrendous inequities we encountered during the course of our work. Some of these offenders have been turned over to the appropriate state agency for prosecution. However, reporting bad doctors is not the primary goal of our group; we are more concerned with teaching people how to avoid dangerous doctors in the first place. It is literally a case of "buyer beware," because your very life may depend on it.

It has become all too common lately that patients entering a hospital to be treated for one disease will end up with another ailment much more serious than the first. This leads us to something called *iatrogenic* disease, which is the technical name now given to health problems caused by doctors. *Iatro* is the Greek word for doctor. Iatrogenic disease is far more widespread than I imagined. Every day thousands of drug side effects and complications during surgery are caused by the kind of medical mistakes I've uncovered. Hospitals are the breeding grounds for iatrogenic problems, because you really can't develop this particular brand of sickness anywhere else. Certainly not at home, where you're a lot safer. Recent studies have revealed that as many as twenty percent of all people who enter American hospitals get iatrogenic disease, and it often results in death. Innumerable patients have developed anemia, heart failure, kidney failure, bizarre infections, liver damage, blindness, bleeding from various bodily sites, lung scarring—all these ailments were contracted *after* they were admitted to the hospital.

Doctors don't like to be reminded of iatrogenic disease. Almost every other disease has its own journal or even a special society, but not this one. And because many doctors and researchers don't focus attention on iatrogenic illness, the public knows little about how to protect against it. That, in our own determined way, is a situation which we at CMQ hope to correct.

Recently, news commentator Paul Harvey stated that autopsies indicate that twenty-four percent of Americans who succumbed to their illnesses were misdiagnosed and ten percent needn't have died at all.

Frequently, unfamiliarity with modern equipment is responsible for this tragedy.

A particularly horrifying example of surgical butchery happened only recently. The perpetrators involved were the very same criminals who had assaulted me—Dr. Kearny and his equally inept colleague, Dr. Robins.

A man in his forties was admitted to the hospital with complaints of severe abdominal pain. He had been under Dr. Robins's care for two weeks prior to admittance, but Robins was still the same careless diagnostician he'd always been, so he kept saying, "Oh, it's probably just a touch of gas."

Finally, on the weekend the man was in such severe pain, he had to be admitted via the hospital's Emergency Room. They got him settled in a room. Dr. Robins came to examine him, and instead of realizing what should have been obvious to him, that the man needed gall bladder surgery at once, Robins followed the usual pattern of his colleagues: he ran the patient through one irrelevant test after the other for the next three days.

It wasn't until the following Wednesday that Dr. Robins decided it was time to operate, but by then the patient's gall bladder was gangrenous. Until that very hour, Robins hadn't even treated the man for this condition. With the ever-careless Dr. Kearny in assistance, the patient was taken to the operating room even though he had a 103-degree temperature.

An elevated temperature indicates infection and if surgery is performed, the infection is spread throughout the body. That is exactly what happened to this poor patient.

The two surgeons began what *should* have been a routine operation, and then it happened: after opening the patient's stomach, Dr. Robins, who was slightly myopic, bent over the man in such an erratic manner that his eye-glasses fell off and landed right in the center of the patient's surgical cavity. From later reports, that scene was so gross, and both surgeons were so rattled by panic, they must have gone a little crazy in their efforts to retrieve the blood-soaked pair of glasses. Sweating and swearing, Dr. Robins, whose vision was now something less than perfect, grabbed a scalpel and tried to flick out the glasses.

In the course of these clumsy efforts, Robins cut up the patient's internal organs so severely that both he and Dr. Kearny were unable to suture the deepening wound. They would barely get him closed up when another opening would appear. They called in their associate, Dr. Butler. He, too, tried to close up the wound, but to no avail.

Finally, the patient was sutured as well as they could manage. Then they put him in the intensive care unit where, at four the next morning, he died of internal bleeding. For once there was no attempt at a coverup or conspiracy. This horror was all over the hospital. The nurses were so outraged they told everyone about it.

One of the nurses was so appalled by this latest atrocity, she documented the whole case for me, and I've turned it over to all the appropriate state agencies. However, it is the victim's wife who must take action in this case. All we can do is pray she won't let these incompetent doctors get away with murder.

Unfortunately, even if this woman does seek justice, medical litigation will drag on for an interminable length of time while in the interim these butchers are permitted to go on doing their worst without so much as a reprimand.

In "real life," if all those people had witnessed such a crime, all they'd have to do is call the police and say, "I saw what those men did—I was in the room with them when they did it," and the two criminals would be arrested at once. But the rarefied milieu that shelters doctors affords them a medical diplomatic immunity which in no way resembles "real life." It is, at the very least, "unreal" that these men are allowed to go on committing the same crimes, year after year.

Chapter Nineteen

I was given the opportunity to help so many people during our first year in business, I hardly know where to begin. There were several reasons for so much swift, word-of-mouth publicity. Although I had always been very social, I did not realize until now how many friends I had in town, and what a surprising number of them supported me in this daring project. For our ultra-conservative area, 'daring' was the right word to describe what I was doing. Things like this simply didn't happen in our town. And if they did, I was the last person anyone expected to be connected with such a controversial project. What nerve I had, to start a medical consumer group in a town where so many doctors were already under investigation (thanks to some of my earlier ground-work).

In the past I had always been such a meek conformist. And while it was true my manner was as meek as ever, my actions proved beyond the shadow of a doubt that I wasn't the girl I used to be.

One of the early results of my publicity was a letter I received from a man whose five-year-old girl had a twenty percent curvature of the spine, or scoliosis. Scoliosis is a lateral (sideways) deviation of the backbone, caused by congenital or acquired abnormalities of the vertebrae, muscle weakness, or nerve disorders. Normally they won't do anything about this condition unless it involves a thirty-percent curvature. After he had her examined in Bay City, they advised him to take her home. At that time they would either go in surgically and correct the curvature or they would implant different types of transmitters, thereby giving the patient a form of shock treatment which would tighten the muscles. On occasion, they would get pretty good results with this method.

The little girl's father wrote me that he had heard of a new treatment involving a medical appliance called the Scolitron. This is an apparatus that is strapped to the child during her sleeping hours, at an age when she is still growing, preferably no older than ten or twelve. This man's little five-year-old was the ideal age for this treatment. It is not painful. Due to the pulsation transmitted via the Scolitron, it actually strengthens muscles. In fact, children using it don't even have their sleep disturbed. This also dispenses with the need to wear a special brace twenty-four hours a day, as this is something the children only wear at night.

Of course, I didn't know any of this until I investigated. Indeed, nobody this man spoke to about it had even heard of it. Nor would they offer to help him or enlighten him further on the subject. Thwarted by the experts, this man had come to me as a last resort.

I researched the problem in my library. Among my many medical journals, I read an article discussing a new kind of treatment that sounded very much like the Scolitron. This research was being conducted by a doctor in southern California. I phoned the center he worked at and was lucky enough to speak directly to this doctor.

He agreed that the Scolitron was one of the new treatments he was researching. "But you should deal directly with the manufacturer," he said. "He's the man you want."

"I couldn't agree with you more, Doctor," I said. "Where do I find him?"

"He's in Texas," he said.

The doctor gave me a toll-free number to call, which I did, as soon as I hung up. Naturally the manufacturer was very cooperative, as they were ready to start marketing this product and agreed it was time the public knew more about it. They sent me all the information about the Scolitron anyone would need, including where and how to order it, the cost, even directions on how to use it. I forwarded all this research to the man and he got the ball rolling on his own. He phoned me several weeks later and told me how grateful he was for the information.

"Chalk one up for our side," I told Steve that night.

The fact that knowledge was power was something I grew more certain of with each new and troubled consumer I was able to enlighten.

I dealt with many people face to face, so often I was able to view the results of my labors. One woman came to see me and, without wasting much time, said, "I just moved here, and I've got a very strange disease. It's called 'polyarteritisnodosa,' and I know you've never heard of it. But the point is, practically any doctor you contact knows all about it. But my doctor never even heard of it. Would you believe it?"

"Does your doctor practice in this area?"

"Yes," she said.

I smiled. "Then I believe it."

She asked if I would dig up some information about this disease, so she could prove to her doctor she wasn't imagining things. When she told me the general area of her body where the symptoms were centered, I immediately thought of an excellent rheumatologist who might be able to help. I called him and asked if I could borrow a book he had on this subject. He and his staff were nice enough to send me more than I asked for, adding up to some extensive information on polyarteritisnodosa. I quickly mailed this to the woman in question and hoped she would use it to prove to her doctor that this disease did, indeed, exist.

Only a few days later, I had to go to the medical library, involved in still another research project. As I sat there, poring over the journals, who should walk in and take a seat at the opposite side of the room but Dr. Post himself. He just gave me a sheepish nod when he came in, though I knew how it annoyed him and his other accomplices to know that one of their surgical mistakes was still alive and well and stirring up trouble.

We sat there in the library for about forty-five minutes, each absorbed in our own research. He read intently from several heavy volumes, making copious notes. That was the first time I had ever seen this man so heavily involved in research, and it got me curious. When he left the library, the librarian mentioned to me that he had been researching information on polyarteritisnodosa.

Now I knew who that woman's doctor was. Dr. Post. And there he was, having to bone up on this disease because, thanks to my help, his patient now knew more about it than he did. I thought that was such a sweet touch of irony: the more I educated the locals, the more on top of things the doctors would have to be.

It was no problem for me to gain access to a medical library that had formerly been reserved for professionals. The first time I went there, I simply told the people in charge about my project and who I was—of course they knew that at first sight—and told them I wanted access to all their research materials as well as their Med-Line computer linkup to the National Institutes of Health at Bethesda, Maryland.

"Of course, Mrs. Carroll," the head librarian said. I pay a nominal fee of ten dollars for using the computer, though the librarian provides this service, after I tell her what I want to know.

It seems to be a fact of history and tradition that any rebel in our midst who stands up and refuses to accept any more corruption and incompetence is regarded as a nonconformist; thus, not to be trusted. If more people had the courage to ask "why?," this wouldn't be such a lonely role to play. The attitude of most patients is that there is no use to complain when they're at the mercy of experts who know so much more about their health than they do.

If they are so convinced that their health care is a *fait accompli*, totally out of their hands, it will only convince the doctors all the more that they really *are* as omnipotent as they'd like to believe.

Yet, since I started my group, I found that more and more of these patients will confide in me, just to unload their grievances. I even get this from some members of the hospital staff. These people know I'm someone who cares, and that I'm neither a political nor a professional threat to them. From the standpoint of hospital workers, they know I'm not after their jobs. As for the worried patients, they know I'm not a doctor, so I'm not competing with whichever doctor happens to be mistreating their particular illness.

Most of all, the patients who came to me were disturbed because their doctors didn't spend more time with them, and refused to treat them with either dignity or respect. After hearing these complaints repeated time and time again, I started speaking to individual doctors, acting as a kind of go-between or advocate between them and their patients.

I might say to the errant doctor, "Now Doctor, this patient is having a hard time communicating with you about her illness, and she's really disturbed by it. Why won't you take the time to listen to her?"

At first, doctors said, "Look, if you're not satisfied with the way I treat you, you can always go to another doctor." Because the area is so insulated and far-removed from other cities, and so many local citizens couldn't afford the cost of driving back and forth to other towns, it used to be a surefire threat when a doctor warned a patient that he might refuse to treat her if she wasn't more agreeable. But lately, due to recent medical aid program cutbacks, as well as the general consumer resistance to high medical costs, doctors all over the state are no longer quite as independent as they used to be, or as quick to send their patients elsewhere if they complain. These doctors live so extravagantly, and their financial responsibilities are so heavy, that their patient-load only has to drop off for a few weeks and they start to feel it where it matters the most, in their wallets.

Naturally, that's one recent development I find very encouraging: the hungrier these men are, the more willing they will be to treat the consumer—the buying public—with the respect and concern they're paying for.

As for the most frequent questions patients ask us, most of them involve a concern about the side effects they might expect from a particular drug. Few of our local doctors will volunteer this kind of information. And because the majority of our average citizens are quiet, unassuming, uneducated, and, in some cases, even illiterate, it would never occur to them to say, "Hey, Doc, will these pills do anything else to me besides what they're supposed to do?" A very simple question, but one that is all too rarely asked.

Luckily, I'm able to give the patients this information, via my research library, provided they have the good sense to come to me with their questions in the first place.

As for the doctors who don't spend enough time with their patients, we have one guy in town who should be listed in the *Guinness Book of Records*. This man will see more than one hundred patients a day, spending an average of five minutes with each patient. He runs a clinic and has eight examining rooms. He flits from room to room, dispensing instant malpractice in each of them, and charges thirty-one dollars per patient. This is a real pill-pusher. I've decided he's either bionic or he runs on supercharged batteries. I'm sure his poor, victimized patients must encounter all the tender loving care they'd find going through a revolving door.

I am so determined to enlighten all these people that I've seriously toyed with the idea of driving my own motorized library from house to house, just to show them that the right information could cure a lot of ailments their doctors might not even be able to diagnose.

Actually, many of the books in my library had been published too recently to have gained the attention of many of the area's esteemed physicians, most of whom spend a lot more time reading the *Wall Street Journal*.

Unfortunately, I have received little cooperation from most of the doctors I've approached on behalf of a patient. They were polite and agreeable, but they were also very noncommittal, offering neither defense nor explanation. Some of them smiled and listened, but I could tell how eager they were to say, "Goodbye, Mrs. Carroll. Have a nice day."

One doctor I spoke to was incredibly nasty. I consulted him on behalf of a terminally ill cancer patient, urging him to take more time with this woman, at least enough time to answer her questions.

"Look, Mrs. Carroll, this 'extra time' you're talking about represents money, and I just don't have the time to answer that old lady's dumb questions."

Although I doubt that it registered on the surface, that remark made me furious. "Need I remind you, Dr. Tinsdale, that you are selling a service, one which happens to be your only product. So you'd better *make* time to treat this patient in a civil manner, or maybe the day will come when time is all you have left." Then, just before I turned and walked out of his office, I remembered to smile and say, "Have a nice day."

When I related that incident to some of my business associates, more than one of them said, "If I ever told my customers I didn't have time to be bothered with them, I'd lose their business fast. And I'd deserve to."

But there are still too many patients who are all too willing to be overwhelmed by their doctors, to the point where they accept without question that a doctor is much busier than the rest of us. It's usually the doctor's own choice how many patients he will see. This "heavy schedule" isn't something that is forced on him. He sets his own fees and his own pace. If he's too busy to see any one patient for more than a few minutes at a time, it's only because of his need to make increasingly more money. So he puts his patients on an assembly-line, at thirty dollars a head. It's like a cattle call. Once again, it's a matter of personal greed supplanting the Hippocratic Oath.

Among some of my most rewarding duties as a consumer advocate is the information I've studied—and later dispensed—regarding the many little-known diseases that are gradually coming to light. These are now referred to as "Orphan Diseases," which means, quite literally, that not enough people are afflicted with them to make the development and marketing of the proper medication a profitable venture for the manufacturers. Thankfully, after President Reagan recently signed the Orphan Bill into law, the situation began to look more promising. Now the long-delayed research in developing these much-needed medications can continue.

Imagine that you had a loved one who might be saved by the right medication, but were told by "the industry" that this medication was no longer on the market. The reason: there was no money in it. In other words, there weren't enough people dying from it to make the sale and distribution of such medication a profitable enterprise.

As for the part our group plays regarding those little-known diseases, after I learned enough about them myself, I made efforts to bring all those afflicted in touch with each other. This way they can view their illness as a shared situation, and will, hopefully, feel less alone or isolated with their crisis. Such rare diseases include hemophilia, cystic fibrosis, sickle-cell anemia, thalassemia, Huntington's disease, and Friedreich's ataxia.

An organization called SHARE consists only of people who have lost newborn babies due to birth defects, crib death, and other infant afflictions. I put the right people in touch with this organization. I also offer this liaison service to another group that deals only with newly recovered mental patients, helping these people share the transition of getting back into the mainstream of society and fighting the stigma of their past.

To be able to do this means I have to keep informed as to which special agencies exist, so that all these isolated people can know there *is* somewhere to go to ease their feelings of hopelessness and alienation. Recently, I learned about another rare disease that was really news to me. This is a genetic neurological disease known as "Joseph's Disease." Oddly enough, it afflicts only pure-blooded Portugese people whose ancestors originated in the Azores, in Portugal. It has only been a few years since the major research was completed, but now there is a Joseph's Foundation, an international organization which is intent on publicizing the nature and symptoms of this disease, so that both patients and doctors can learn to diagnose it.

Like our group, all these special agencies are nonprofit corporations, in business only to serve and educate the public.

One day, purely by accident, I discovered another dire need our group was designed to provide. It happened when I visited an elderly resident in a local convalescent home. I had been doing some medical research for Mr. Woodward, so I had reason to visit him on several occasions. Each time I visited him, I noticed that he kept this little box on his lap, as if it contained something very precious to him.

Finally, my curiosity got the better of me and I asked him. "Why is that little box so important to you?"

"Oh, this," he said with a wan smile. He opened it up, and I saw there were about eight little cards and letters inside the box. "These are from my friends and family."

He started reading them aloud for me, then invited me to read a few of them with him. As I did, I saw that some of the cards and letters were years old. I eyed him thoughtfully. "Mr. Woodward, do you get much mail?"

"No," he said with a sigh, "not really."

I thought that was rather sad, the way he held on to old mail, and the fact that he hadn't received any for so long. That got me to wondering how many people there were like him, spending their reclining years in rest homes, all but forgotten by their friends and relatives. I thought how wonderful it would be if there were some way for us to remind all those people that their elderly relatives were still alive and lonely and needed to hear from them. I was sure that a lot of those people had simply lost contact with their old friends, and others had no idea where to reach them. I was also fairly certain there had to be a lot of other people who didn't even know an old friend, or perhaps an uncle, was in a rest home, and

131

that once this was made clear to them, they would phone or write or even pay them a visit.

I kept thinking about this later that night, until an answer suddenly dawned on me while Steve and I were having dinner.

"Greeting cards!" I exclaimed. "That's how we'll do it. Yes, we'll buy cards for the patients to send out to all those people who've forgotten them. Then we'll sit back and wait for the backlash . . . !"

Steve stared at me. "Honey, I'm sure if you run that by me again, I'll be even more confused. But try me anyway."

Then I gave him a complete rundown of exactly what I had in mind, which involved a new form of communication for these patients, and apparently one that nobody had ever thought of before. And thus was born another feature of Consumers For Medical Quality, Inc.: our Greeting Card Project.

After Steve listened carefully to my plan, he smiled and said, "You know, Paula, you never see a problem. You only see the solution."

I looked at him solemnly and said, "Oh Steve, I certainly hope so!"

Chapter Twenty

First, of course, I had to make sure the residents in all of our local convalescent homes might enjoy being able to send greeting cards to long-lost friends or relatives. For this project, I enlisted the aid of Carol Latimer, a good friend of mine who had been going through a medical calamity of her own and was desperately in need of a worthy diversion.

The response from the local homes was overwhelming. Our next chore was a research job: collecting the names and addresses of each patient's relatives, as well as itemizing which birthdays, anniversaries, and holidays they wanted to remember. Then we set out to acquire all the cards we would need, as donations from local stationers, variety stores, and friends. These were surplus cards that had never been sold or used. I then went to some friends who donated money to buy stamps. All the people who made these contributions were as excited as we were about bringing a new dimension to the lives of these shut-ins, and everywhere I heard the same question: "Why didn't anyone think of this before?"

Once we had enough merchandise, Carol and I went to the homes with a large assortment of cards to choose from. We showed them the cards, and they made their choice. These people had become so passive, and were so used to having things done for them, I felt this would give them a chance to reach out on their own, making an affirmative gesture in a new and unexpected way. Later we obtained pledges from other stores for the donation of an unlimited number of cards. We also kept a file for each resident to remind them where cards had already been sent.

We inserted little notes of explanation inside each card, identifying our group and letting the recipients know that this is a free service we're providing for their elderly friends and relatives.

Judging by the response, we must have stirred up a lot of guilt after those hordes of greeting cards arrived at their far-flung destinations. As I had suspected, many of these people had completely lost touch with their elderly friends and relatives, while others had no idea they were even in rest homes. How rewarding it was to see those lonely old people reap their harvest. They began getting lots of mail and cards and Christmas presents and, most important of all, in-person visits from people they hadn't seen in years. After a few months, our novel idea caught on in other areas, and I was even invited to get it started with an out-of-state church group which boasts a membership of ten thousand. Like any good idea, it means so much more when you spread it around. And to think, all it took was a little communication between people who had simply forgotten how much they needed each other.

My friend and helper in this project, Carol Latimer, desperately needed a new outlet at this time because about six months earlier she'd been in an auto accident and had suffered a serious back injury. However, she was a lot more victimized by her doctors than she was by her original injury.

After first being treated at a pain clinic, they took her off her medication and told her they were sending her home, where they had transferred her case to a Dr. Warden, without even asking Carol's opinion of their choice. She and Dr. Warden clashed at their first meeting.

When she told Warden she needed to continue with the pain medication she'd been getting at the pain clinic, the doctor telephoned her prescription into a local pharmacy. As it happened, there was some kind of a mixup: apparently Carol had gotten one final prescription from her pain doctor at the same pharmacy. When the druggist was unable to reach Dr. Warden to verify the prescription, instead of waiting, he simply phoned Carol's former doctor. Knowing that Carol was now being handled by another doctor, this first doctor called Dr. Warden and asked why Carol still had to get her pain prescriptions from him. "I took it for granted that you would be issuing all her prescriptions from now on, Dr. Warden."

"I am," said Warden, "and, in fact, I did." Then he thought about it for a moment and said, "I think I know what's going on here. I'll be in touch with you."

Without even confronting Carol in person, Warden quickly assumed that she was trying to get two prescriptions filled, thereby doubling the amount that he had legitimately prescribed. The medication was empirin with codeine, so Warden took it for granted he had another drug-abuser on his hands.

Warden made his unsubstantiated suspicions official in a letter he wrote to Carol's former doctor. As a result, both doctors were so certain she was getting double prescriptions—and undoubtedly in several pharmacies, not just one—they agreed that Warden should cut back her supply of this medication.

Carol was shattered by this treatment and totally mystified as to what had caused it. She only knew she was still having a great deal of pain. Warden was prescribing less than one-fourth of the amount she needed, without even explaining his reasons. Now she faced the double crisis of her physical condition plus the mental anguish due to Warden's treatment of her. After several months, she became reclusive and deeply depressed. I counseled her during this period and tried to work with her, though I was also at a total loss to understand why she was being persecuted in this manner.

Getting her involved in our Greeting Card Project was a real godsend for Carol. I let her take it over completely, and it proved to be just the reawakening she needed. But in the meantime, I was still trying to solve the mystery, and I knew I wouldn't be satisfied until I had cleared it up.

Luckily, an historic date was coming up and, as it happened, not a minute too soon. On January 1, 1983 it became law: every patient in the state had the right to see his records. Now, I thought, Carol and I can get to the bottom of this. Like many others, it came as a total surprise to Carol when I informed her of her rights. And like her, there are still too many people who don't know anything about this new law, taking it for granted that it's still their doctor who has all the rights in their relationship. I analyzed the situation and decided the problem could be cleared up by a lot of publicity. Our group would certainly start blowing that horn the loudest.

I gave Carol the proper forms to fill out. She went to Dr. Warden's office and had no problem getting her records. She and I went over the file together, and it was then that we found a copy of the letter Dr. Warden had written in which he'd accused her of lying and conspiring to get double prescriptions. After eight long months, this was the first time she knew why those doctors had treated her so cruelly.

"Good grief," she said, "why didn't they just ask me? I was accused without the benefit of making an explanation."

To me it seemed incredible that Warden would write such a letter without taking the trouble to verify his accusations. But most degrading of all, he didn't even respect Carol enough to face her and ask her if his suspicions were correct.

Carol's next step was to go to the pharmacy and get a complete accounting of all her prescriptions. She and the druggist checked this together, and not once was there a duplication recorded. Why hadn't Dr. Warden had the presence of mind to do this same sort of investigation before he jumped to his demeaning conclusion?

Carol confronted Dr. Warden with the records of the pharmacy, plus the copy of his letter to her previous doctor. "This not only proves that you accused me unjustly, but also that you've deliberately denied me the amount of medication I needed, though you knew I was in pain."

Carol told me later that Warden didn't even bat an eyelash. The topper, however, was that Warden sent Carol a bill for that last "visit," as his parting shot. But Carol said she "returned the gesture in tiny bits and pieces."

"Do you think he'll sue?" she joked.

Dr. Warden's reckless and insulting behavior, wherein he was so quick to believe the worst of Carol without bothering to substantiate his accusations, pretty much reflects the attitude of many doctors: *when in doubt, the patient is always wrong.*

If these men make it so clear they have no respect for their patients, how can they be expected to care enough to make them well? Or, more importantly, is it possible for this kind of contempt and the practice of good medicine to go hand in hand? Just thinking about such a contradiction in terms is more than a little unsettling—and very scary.

The need for our special services continued to grow. I had, and needed, more volunteer help in my home-office. This came in handy when I got launched on my speaking engagements, which took me all over the state. Although this would mark my debut in "show business," I knew instinctively that I couldn't sound as intense or keyed-up about some of these inequities as I personally felt. I had to remember to remain cool and detached while discussing the activities of our consumer group. This was also true when I related some of the medical horror stories to which I had been exposed. This way, I could leave it to my audiences to become emotionally disturbed, while I told them these facts like a concerned professional, not a ranting agitator.

I spoke at colleges, service clubs, women's groups, and church groups, editing my material to suit each audience. I would tell them about my library, our various services, or I might discuss a particularly disturbing case of medical abuse, so they might empathize with these statistics as flesh-and-blood human victims. Because I have such a wealth of information to share, I find that the more I learn, the more "news" I have to impart to each new group I see.

In June of 1982, it was due to my concern over a troubled cancer patient that I got the idea to add still another vital service to our consumer group—CMQ's Emergency Fund. But first let me tell you something about the woman who inspired this worthy project.

Her name was Muriel Watson. She was hospitalized with what I later learned was inoperable lung cancer. She told me she wanted to see me, that she needed some important advice. When I first started talking to her, at her bedside, I assumed that all she wanted to know was how to go about demanding a second opinion.

"That's very simple," I told her. "The next time your doctor comes to see you, you tell him—and notice, I said 'tell' not 'ask'—that you want to go for a second opinion." Then, because she was in a hospital I knew all too well, I got curious. "Who is your doctor, by the way?"

"Dr. Post."

It wasn't easy, but I kept my "poker face." Of course, my first instinct was to wheel her out to safety without saying another word. But I had learned to be subtle and diplomatic when it came to judging the criminals of my past.

"Post," I said, mulling this over. "But he's a surgeon."

"Oh yes, I know," she said. Then she went on to tell me about the extensive surgery she'd just had, though now she wanted a second opinion. I knew she had lung cancer, and I had a feeling she was going for that second opinion a bit late. Admittedly, the fact that Post is well known for doing unnecessary surgery got me very suspicious. Along with his manic ego-drive, shared with so many of his surgical colleagues, Post also shared their favorite credo: "When in doubt, cut it out."

"Are you sure they didn't just do a biopsy?" I asked her.

"Oh no. They did that earlier. Then they did this other operation."

"After the biopsy, did they say if the lymph nodes were positive?"

"Yes," she said, "they did."

That's when I was certain that they had done nothing but some needless exploratory surgery on this woman. They knew from the results of the biopsy that her lung cancer was inoperable, because it had spread to the area behind the lung known as the mediastinum.[1] I sat there thinking: this day and age, even if such surgery had been indicated, there would have been no need for it, due to the many new alternatives available, any of which an enlightened surgeon would have preferred to simply cutting the patient up for no reason at all.

I was concentrating so intently, and had remained silent for so long, Mrs. Watson must have sensed my concern.

"He said I would die if I didn't have it," she said.

"Pardon?"

"Dr. Post," she said. "He was so angry with me when I first refused the surgery. He yelled at me and said I'd only live two months if I didn't consent to the surgery. He gave me no choice. And my family—my brother and sister—they think I should go up to Bay City Medical Center and get some more answers."

"So do I, Mrs. Watson," I said. "And the sooner the better."

Actually, only about twenty-five percent of lung cancer cases are discovered in time to be operable, because it's so long before any overt symptoms can be felt.[2] By the time these warning signs are evident, it's too late for an operation to help.

Later, when Mrs. Watson was treated by the number one surgeon at Bay City Medical Center, he examined Post's earlier x-ray, and, in the presence of the patient's sister and brother, he said, "I don't understand. Post must have known by looking at this x-ray that he could accomplish absolutely nothing by going in there. I mean, it's very clear to me that this tumor is inoperable."

"Are you telling us the doctor did unnecessary surgery on our sister?" Mrs. Watson's brother asked.

The doctor looked at him. "Yes, frankly, that's exactly what he did. But it wouldn't do for you to alienate that man, not if you planned to get further medical treatment when you go home."

He was implying, unfortunately, that these people had no alternative. Because Post was the only doctor handling Mrs. Watson's case, they couldn't afford to get him angry at her. "You'll still be a patient in that hospital, under his care," he added, "so you don't want to make an enemy of him."

With everything else this woman now had to contend with, to be given such an outrageous warning about the only doctor she could go home to must have intensified all her fears and anxieties. And yet, Mrs. Watson was destitute, so she had nowhere else to go but home.

Muriel Watson was a divorcee who had worked as a secretary for a small, independent business. Many such offices with fewer than five workers do not have employee hospitalization insurance, so that was another strike Muriel had against her: no insurance.

Originally, I helped Muriel and her brother when they first planned to drive up to Bay City. Her brother had never driven in the city before, so I gave them some tips, and also got them a reservation in Bay City so they

138

could stay overnight. When she insisted on financing this on her own, I said, "The *CMQ Emergency Fund* will take care of it."

She and her brother gave me a look of surprise.

"I didn't know you people had your own emergency fund," said her brother.

Neither did I, actually, but as it turned out, I didn't waste much time in making that wishful thought come true. "Oh, we've been keeping it under wraps until now," I told them. "But you just watch and see how much publicity we're going to give it."

If anyone needed such help, it was Muriel Watson. She had no dependents and lived by herself. Her brother and sister had large families of their own and were heavily in debt. Aside from having no medical insurance, the fact that she had no dependents meant that she didn't qualify for welfare either, so she fell through the cracks of all our social programs. It was true that she had qualified for medical welfare to pay for the surgery already performed, but she was no longer able to earn the money she'd need to feed and clothe herself, or pay her rent and utilities, much less provide the medication and vitamins she would need. As if that weren't enough, when she got back to town, she only had twenty-four dollars left in her checking account.

Muriel's predicament made me realize the important service that had been missing in our group—emergency loans for the desperate. As I well knew, it was a big enough battle to struggle with a terminal disease under the best of conditions, when there's enough money for everything. But not to have money for shelter, food, and medicine at a time like this is a burden no terminal patient should have to contend with.

That's exactly how I put it to Steve that night when I told him about Muriel Watson. I was certain there must be many others like her, people with life-threatening diseases who are also destitute.

"So, what do you think? I want to create an emergency loan fund as part of CMQ's activities."

He gave me a playful grin, but I knew that he knew I was serious. "Does the Salvation Army know about you?"

"No, this won't be charity," I said. "It will be done in the form of a loan. I've figured it all out: most people in need find it a lot easier to accept a loan than charity. And if it's given as a loan, it won't interfere with anyone's eligibility for other forms of assistance; you know, like welfare or whatever. And besides, the person given a loan can look forward to being able to pay it back, which gives him a goal and adds to his self-esteem. It'll also give him a more positive attitude about recovering from his illness. What do you think about it?"

"I like it," he said. Indeed, he liked it so much, that this time he insisted on getting in on the act. He enlisted the aid of our good friend, the former FBI investigator, Fred Augustine, as well as several other business associates. That weekend we got a committee together, then called our banker and told him we would be in on Monday morning to set up the fund. When Monday morning rolled around, we all got together and did just that. After we got all the legal aspects ironed out with our accountant and our attorney, I decided to go out and get some local publicity. Because this was a story about helping the destitute, rather than an exposé on the local doctors, I felt sure no local newspaper would find it too "controversial" to touch.

As it turned out, I was right. The reporter I gave the story to did a beautiful job on it, mentioning our group and the new emergency fund, urging readers who wanted to make donations to send the money to our bank. This caught on so quickly, it was astounding. In less than three weeks we had raised about eight thousand dollars.

During that first week, I decided to have a garage sale. I did not take the time to first figure out exactly what I had to sell. Not very much, as it turned out—I only had eight little bags of articles. And our garage was so big. "Oh well," I said to Steve, "we can always sell the garage."

But, as it happened, I had a lot of help. From neighborhood contributions, we filled up more than just our garage. We had to branch out and take over one of the biggest vacant stores in town. The result was a financial triumph. We made over sixteen hundred dollars in just two days. We had so many items left over, we donated the overflow to the Salvation Army, and that gave us all an extra lift.

That sixteen hundred dollars represented our first loan. It went to Muriel Watson, of course. When I told her about the success of our efforts, she broke down and cried, telling me how ashamed she was. But I talked her out of keeping it a secret, convincing her how it would help publicize the fund and also lead the way for others if she let her story be told in the local newspaper. Later, thanks to continued donations to the fund, we were able to pay Muriel's rent, food, utilities, and by then we were also supporting two other patients who were destitute and had no other resources. Many were happy to contribute, as all donations are tax deductible and one hundred percent of the money goes to those who need it. No overhead or expense accounts are paid out of the fund.

None of the people borrowing this money are charged interest, and their repayment plan is based only on their sufficient recovery and ability to return to work. Eventually, our maximum loan was fixed at 450 dollars per month, for a maximum period of ninety days. But because Muriel was the forerunner of this project, and she was good enough to go public with her story, we contributed to her support as long as she needed it. She died nine months later.

Incidentally, despite the warning about not alienating Dr. Post, Muriel couldn't bring herself to go back to him again. She felt safer at home, in her own bed, now that she knew what might befall her if she were again under Post's jurisdiction. Later, she became desperately ill at home and her sister phoned me at six in the morning and said Muriel was spitting up blood.

Dr. Post was still Muriel's physician of record, and in our town it was always risky to hope that some other doctor would be willing to take over. Fortunately, by now I knew the most competent and trustworthy doctors in town.

Despite the early morning hour, I called one of them. I told him about Muriel and her illness, and her terminal prognosis. Then I told him about Muriel's emergency at the moment. "Can you see her, Dr. Hughes?"

"All these months post-op with terminal lung cancer? Mrs. Carroll, if this woman has been seeing another doctor, you must know what a difficult position you're putting me in."

"We're talking about Muriel Watson's position at the moment, Dr. Hughes, and it sounds as if she is hemorrhaging. What she needs is instant help, not a discussion of medical politics."

"Who was her previous doctor?"

"I don't understand all of the problems. But she needs a doctor now."

"Okay, tell her to call me after nine. I'll make arrangements to see her in my office some time today."

When I hung up, I was about to try another doctor who would take some action immediately. But Dr. Hughes called me right back. "Mrs. Carroll, I've reconsidered. I'll meet the patient at the hospital emergency room within the hour."

"Thank you, Doctor. That's all I wanted to hear."

Dr. Hughes was affiliated with the same hospital where Dr. Post still performed his feats of bungling, and I could only speculate as to what sort of conflicts these two physicians had when Muriel Watson was admitted to the hospital and made it clear that she had "fired" her original doctor.

[1] Medical literature on this point is quite specific, as seen in the following quotes:

"Exploration (surgery) can often be avoided when metastases are demonstrated by mediastinoscopy." —Berkow, ed., *Merck Manual*, 14th edition, Rahway, NJ: Merck, 1982, p. 697.

"Operations for lung cancer are major surgery and are usually not performed unless the patient stands a reasonable chance for cure." —Morra and Potts, *Choices: Realistic alternatives in cancer treatment*, New York: Avon, 1980, p. 330.

"Surgery should only be done if there is no evidence of spread of the cancer beyond the lung." —Glucksberg and Singer, *Cancer Care: a personal guide*, New York: Scribner's, 1982, p. 338.

[2] "Only about 25% of the tumors are resectable." —Berkow, ed., *Merck Manual*, 14th edition, Rahway, NJ: Merck, 1982, p. 697.

Chapter Twenty-one

*A*side from the varied "humanity services" our group provides, we kept fighting the good fight for some very necessary legal reforms, though it appeared that several existing laws would have to be changed before we succeeded in this battle.

In 1984, for example, economists announced that 400 billion dollars were spent for medical health care, fifty percent of which came from the taxpayers. Yet the taxpayer has nothing to say about how that money is spent or how the health care is dispensed. Why are we so content to be silent partners in a process that is costing us so much of our hard-earned money?

Often on state board review committees there are only two laypersons pitted against six doctors. What kind of representation is that? I feel I've proved that if he's sufficiently motivated, any layperson can become informed enough to determine the quality of his own health care. If we "average" consumers were as uninformed as the experts try to make us believe, we wouldn't be such a threat to them. Yet we must pose a threat to them; why else would they go to such great lengths to keep laypersons off state boards and committees and continue to conduct secret meetings? I don't think it's because we wouldn't understand. On the contrary, it's because we would.

It seems so archaic that there is still this "traditional" reluctance on the part of the medical community to share its secrets with the public. How can they fail to realize that people are simply more informed these days, due to the media and the many published exposés on the inequities so prevalent in the doctor-patient relationship? Instead, they seem to dwell in a kind of perennial time warp, clinging to their long-obsolete gentlemen's agreements and their double standards. Some of these dinosaurs still believe they shouldn't be sued if they make an honest mistake. Can you imagine a building contractor or an engineer offering that same lame excuse if one of his "honest mistakes" causes a wall or a bridge to collapse, resulting in death and injuries? Why should the physician be exempt from the same moral responsibility?

Luckily, CMQ found a great ally—and I found a perceptive confidante—in the person of Dave Callisher, one of the top officials with MSB. In my case, this association was tantamount to having a friend at court.

Dave Callisher was very tuned-in to the epidemic of medical abuse. Recently he said to me, "Paula, let me know whenever a patient signs a complaint against a doctor. Then I can get the records from the hospital before the doctor has a chance to clean them up." He was referring, of course, to the altering, falsifying, and sometimes total revision of the medical records.

The state's Health Service Agency was set up during the sixties, when there was so much over-building and so many duplicate services being foisted on the public. The Agency was established in order to restrict the way in which money was spent for equipment or new facilities. According to this law, doctors or hospital administrators were required to produce a Certificate of Need, proving their proposed expansion was justified before they were given the money to finance it.

Dave Callisher told me that most doctors have long since found a way to get around that law. They simply rent whatever new equipment they want from companies which they, the doctors, own, and which they manipulate to show a perpetual loss.

Many doctors have also learned how to "juggle" their malpractice premiums the same way. For example, a doctor pays thirty thousand dollars a year for this insurance, and during that year he doesn't have any actions filed against him. He will then have built up a credit with his insurance company, which will be returned to him in the form of dividends, retirement funds, or even a life insurance policy. By doing this, he is inadvertently driving up the cost of malpractice insurance. And though these payments have nothing to do with malpractice, the doctor is the one who benefits. These men find so many ways to finagle and reroute their flow of income, it's a wonder they have time for anything else. When they complain, "I'm spending thirty thousand dollars a year for malpractice insurance," they overlook the fact that they can actually be making an investment for themselves, a "cushion fund" they can fall back on later.

Such doctors are so bogged down in bookkeeping and paperwork, as well as the protocol and administrative duties of the institution, that they've come to consider an interruption from a mere patient to be something of a nuisance, even irrelevant. They forget that it was the needs of these patients that put them in their profession in the first place. Now they have totally reversed their priorities by avoiding the patient; they prefer to spend their time figuring out their capital gains or their tax shelters.

Recently, a local man told me of an experience he'd had with a doctor who was as tactless as he was greedy.

"I was in the middle of a complete physical exam," he said. "It was winter and very cold in the doctor's treatment room. Everything went along fine until suddenly, while I was still standing there naked, the doctor's phone rang. He didn't even say 'excuse me.' He picked it up and I could tell at once that he was talking to his stockbroker. He jabbered on and on about buying this, selling that, doing this with his shares of IBM and that with his shares of AT&T. As the minutes ticked by, I was getting colder and colder. I couldn't believe what was happening. He was selling short and I was turning blue! It was as if he'd forgotten I was alive. Now I ask you, how can you forget a tubby, middle-aged man who is standing totally naked only a few feet away from you? For a minute he had me thinking I'd become invisible.

"Finally, I had enough. I went over, tapped him on the shoulder, and said loud enough for his broker to hear, 'Listen, Doctor, I'm standing here naked and I'm freezing to death waiting for you to remember what business you're in. So unless you want to treat me for pneumonia, hang up the damned phone!' Well, that man gave me such a stunned look, you'd think he'd never laid eyes on me before. Stammering something into the phone, he hung up. Then he told me he was sorry, but I should understand it was an important call. 'It was long distance,' he said. And I said, 'The hell with long distance, what about *my* longevity? That's what you should be concerned with right now. That's why you're here and that's what I'm paying you for. Now if that comes as too much of a shock to you, I'll put my clothes on and take my business elsewhere!' Which, I'm glad to report, I finally did."

That delightful story, which was almost too true to be funny, proved that not all patients are too intimidated by their doctors to fight back whenever the need arises. If only more patients had that kind of righteous indignation. Perhaps then our doctors wouldn't be so quick to dismiss us as inferior merchandise, simply because we didn't spend as much money on our education as they did. Of course, in many cases they haven't cracked a medical book since getting their diploma thirty or forty years ago.

Unfortunately, the patient rebellion mentioned above is all too rare. Ironically enough, the reverse is true. For some unfathomable reason, no matter how a doctor may foul up, there will always be those diehard patients who insist on remaining loyal to him, even after all the evidence has been weighed and the doctor in question may have lost his license.

This actually happened in the case of a doctor who has been called "an absolute menace," even by his own colleagues. He was caught selling narcotics to his patients, stripped of his license, convicted of a felony, and actually served a jail term. When he was released, I was amazed to hear how all his friends and former patients were rallying around this man, demanding that his license be restored. Here was a man who actually did time for pushing drugs, and all these supposedly "sane" people still wanted him to be their doctor.

When I discussed this case with Dave Callisher, he said, "Obviously, this guy came from a nice background, had an attractive manner, a winning personality. With some people, that's all that matters. They're able to judge his charming behavior, but they are not in a position to judge his medical expertise. Therefore, I guess they only rely on what they're able to understand."

Initially I took exception to that comment, feeling most patients aren't nearly educated enough to know how they're being victimized. But later I had to admit that if a patient continues to defend substandard treatment even after the facts are made known, then he does, indeed, deserve what he gets. True, I feel the public has a right to know in advance if a doctor they're planning to see is dangerous or untrustworthy. But if he still chooses to see that man after he's been duly warned, then all responsibility for what might happen to that patient is strictly his own concern.

Still, this continues to be one of the vital services we provide at CMQ. When someone calls and asks us to recommend a doctor they can trust, we have a very handy list on file, notable mostly for the names that are *not* listed. Actually, there exists no other surefire system whereby a person who might be new to a city can contact an agency who will recommend the best doctor available. Usually, if they call the state medical society or the AMA, they will either recommend the first three doctors on the list, or they'll "push" the newest doctors just starting out, in an effort to help them get started. Granted, that's a lot of help to the doctors, but absolutely no use to the unsuspecting patient.

If a patient tells me he plans to see Drs. Kearny, Post, Butler, Forbes, or Robins, I have to be careful not to say anything libelous at the mere utterance of those names. Instead, I simply say, "You can pass over that one...and that one...." I'll wait until they mention someone I know can

146

help them. For example, if they mention Forbes, I won't hesitate to recommend him. True, I have reason to know this man doesn't have both oars in the water, but by local standards, he's still one of the best doctors in the area.

There are times when I am called on to counsel the relatives of terminal patients. In one case a man phoned me and said the wife of a good friend of his was being treated in a hospital and was dying of inoperable lung cancer. This man's friend was devastated, and needed some reliable reassurance that his wife was getting the best treatment available. This means so much to the grieving survivors, just to have the satisfaction of knowing that all that can possibly be done *is* being done.

I drove to see him, and as I knew his wife was definitely in the best of hands in that hospital, I spoke to this man for over an hour. Due to my own experience with cancer, plus all the research I had done on the subject, when he told me the details of his wife's treatment, I knew that what was being done for her was good medicine. I also knew that this hospital was in constant touch with the doctors at Bay City, who readily shared their research and expertise with them. I discussed all this with the grieving man and assured him his wife was being handled by the right professionals at the right time.

I could see how much this reassurance meant to him. If he'd had any doubts about her treatment, or discovered later that he could have done better for her, after her death he would have suffered a heavy guilt trip, and he would forever ask himself, "Did I do all I could for her?" But now, after our talk, he knew he would have nothing for which to reproach himself. And, not incidentally, that also gave me a very good feeling, knowing I had the ability to extend comfort to someone so distraught at a time like that.

The more well-known I became as a medical advocate, the more respect I received from many of the officials at the MSB. Through my efforts, in only a year we managed to send in about twenty-five signed complaints to MSB, which was more than they had ever received in such a short space of time.

On the other hand, it remains very uncertain as to what will be done with those complaints once they've been filed. Due to the bureaucratic foul-ups wrought by these state agencies, whereby they are slowly permitting the medical community to dominate their thinking, agencies like MSB will never become consumer-oriented as long as the majority of physicians are considerably more affluent than their average patients. Unfortunately, money is power, the kind of power that still talks where it matters the most—at the board meetings of top state officials.

The following further illustrates how some doctors are in danger of being consumed by their own greed. One doctor who earns more than 200 thousand dollars a year recently tried to get a bank loan, but was turned down. The bank managers considered him a bad risk: if he couldn't hack it on 200 thousand dollars a year, how could he manage the necessary loan payments?

Doctors like these, who are under such pressure to maintain an extravagant lifestyle, often resort to the habit of over-billing to compensate for the gap in their cash flow. Recently a patient came to me complaining about a doctor, Albert Mendoza, who had ripped her off while she was hospitalized.

"He would poke his head in my hospital room for just a minute or two," she said. "He'd say 'Hi there, how are you today?' Then he would disappear and bill me for a fifty-dollar hospital visit. And the thing is, he's not even my doctor."

This was a new one, even to *my* ears. "Well, maybe your own doctor asked him to check in on you."

"No, he didn't, Mrs. Carroll. I asked him, and he said 'Certainly not. I didn't ask that doctor to see you.' "

I suggested she file an official complaint. It was obvious this doctor was simply hustling up more money, relying on the gullibility of most patients, certain that none of them would even question his door-to-door thievery. But when this woman filed her complaint with Medicare, they replied that there was no merit to her case. The reason: her own doctor had reversed his statement when questioned by the authorities, saying, in effect, "Yes, I did authorize this doctor to look in after my patient." When the patient insisted that he had said exactly the opposite to her, the doctor flatly denied it.

I found this so outrageous, I decided to question this decision, in person, with a Medicare public relations executive who, as luck would have it, just happened to be in Bay City at the same time I was. By this time I had already gone through the proper Medicare channels, with nothing to show for my efforts except the same old pass-the-buck evasions, platitudes, and bureaucratic red tape.

I had documented proof that this doctor was overcharging patients, some of whom he'd never even seen before he poked his head in their room for a fifty-dollar "visit."

"In effect, this doctor uses the hospital corridors as if they were a bunch of Las Vegas slot machines," I said. "He just goes from door to door, hoping he'll get lucky. I guess he figures that two or three jackpots per floor can really make his day."

The executive, whose name was Richmond, seemed amused by this comparison, but he was also genuinely sympathetic. Of course, it wasn't sympathy I was looking for—it was action.

"Actually, most gamblers are better losers than the men you're talking about, Mrs. Carroll. Doctors like these can't afford to lose, not with the kind of expenditures they have to deal with. So they do what most crooks do when they want to support an expensive habit—they steal."

He also told me there was no way to prosecute the average doctor who overbills. "Let's say a doctor admits that he's giving a patient a minimum visit, which should cost about fifteen dollars. Such a visit should only entail about three to five minutes. But he can easily put that down as a comprehensive visit, in which case he might charge seventy-five dollars or one hundred dollars. Who's to say the visit wasn't 'comprehensive?' This is between the doctor and the patient, who is rarely informed enough to know the difference. This is the sort of Medicare fraud we're watching out for now. In fact, the State's Attorney's office is also investigating the matter.

"Unfortunately, we can only prosecute the really greedy ones. In fact, out of the thousands of cases that come to us each year, last year we were only able to prosecute twenty of them."

Another "scam" is run by most doctors, especially those whose credo is "You Fill My Pockets, I'll Fill Yours." One such complaint involved five or six doctors, all working for the same clinic. The way it works is that a patient will go to the clinic and get a first diagnosis from Dr. X. But Dr. X says, "I can't make a positive diagnosis, so I'm going to call in a colleague of mine, Dr. Y."

Dr. Y looks at the patient, but says he's not sure either, so he calls in another colleague. This is a conspiracy going on here: these "good buddies" want to make sure that as many of them as possible get a piece of this pie. Not only is this blatant fraud, it is also a waste of the patient's valuable time. Instead of being given the correct diagnosis as quickly as possible, treatment is delayed long enough for five or six "consulting" doctors to bill their eighty-dollar fee for assisting with a case where only one physician was needed.

All this is set in motion by the primary physician, who, in most cases, knows what's wrong with the patient without having to call in anyone else. This is being done all the time, and it's a crime that will continue as long as patients refuse to question such suspicious behavior.

Similar complaints involve doctors who make hospital calls at midnight, at a time when they know the patient is asleep. They claim they don't want to waken the patient for an actual visit, but they charge for a visit just the same, billing the patient for a routine hospital call of which he was never aware.

Dr. Albert Mendoza, the above-mentioned doctor who went from room to room, "visiting" patients who were not even assigned to him, was by far the greediest hustler in town. He alone had the gall to bill a patient for a visit a full twenty-four hours after that patient had died and had been wheeled to the morgue. And Mendoza did this more than once, though we'll get into more of this man's crimes later.

The fact that the deceased patient's heirs never questioned such billing only proves that the need for patient education grows more desperate every year. Surely, the more "aware in advance" each consumer becomes, the less likely it will be that these blatant frauds can continue.

Chapter Twenty-two

*D*r. Albert Mendoza was a physician from Costa Rica who was at the center of an incredibly heated controversy. After countless complaints that Mendoza was practicing poor medicine and ordering too many needless—and expensive—tests for his patients, many of whom were low-income blue collar workers on welfare, Dr. Forbes, chairman of the Emergency Room Committee, started proceedings to have Mendoza stripped of his staff privileges. Among many other complaints, Forbes accused Mendoza of performing too many unneeded "diagnostic procedures," which tied up needed space in the hospital.

To retaliate, Dr. Mendoza ended up suing the hospital, claiming he was the target of a vendetta by other physicians who were not only losing business to him, but were also racially prejudiced against him. Sadly, only about ten or fifteen percent of the hospital personnel wanted to oust Mendoza. Most of the nurses felt that ninety-five percent of the hospital's problems would disappear if they got rid of Dr. Mendoza. But the bottom line was in Mendoza's favor: he put his patients through so many expensive tests and procedures, he generated a lot of extra income for the hospital. It didn't matter to the administrators that most of those procedures were totally unnecessary. As long as he made money for "the team," they wanted him to remain.

And so the war began. And with it, the dirty infighting between those members of the staff who favored Mendoza and those who wanted him to leave the hospital staff.

Dr. Post, one of Mendoza's supporters, knew how much extra money this man was bringing in, so he filed a complaint against Dr. Forbes, reporting him to MSB for certain "inequities," simply because Forbes had launched the original complaint against Mendoza. Further retaliation followed, creating an aura of malice and childish duplicity that more accurately reflected the atmosphere in a boys' reformatory than that of a group of grown medical practitioners.

Upon learning of Post's reports to MSB, Mendoza's enemies pressured a patient who had been fouled up by Mendoza—only one of many—to sue the offending doctor. This was to be their revenge against Post and Mendoza for reporting Dr. Forbes and his followers to MSB. Dr. Post then tried to persuade a family to sue Dr. Forbes.

It seems incredible to think of all those petty ego games being played in a major hospital, while the needs of the patients were all but forgotten. Indeed, there was such widespread paranoia and suspicion among the doctors as a result of this war, that another doctor started building a seven-foot brick and wrought iron fence around his estate, while Dr. Mendoza, who said his life had been threatened, posted armed security guards outside his home. Perhaps they were expecting an uprising from those patients who had managed to survive the treatment they'd been given by doctors like Mendoza, Post, Robins, Kearny, and Dr. Chad Cowgill.

It was during this period that the figure of the Godfather emerged. It was none other than Dr. Cowgill. His word was law and he got things done...his way. He had enormous charisma and wealth to match it.

By observing the "pecking order" within the system, it seemed this Dr. Cowgill was some kind of a feudal lord. He commanded homage just because of his very "presence." He seemed to believe that in order to succeed he had to be manipulative and earn *a lot* of money, rather than be a good doctor. When the other doctors spoke of him it was with awe and misplaced respect.

All this added tension created spinoff feuds between the doctors' wives, many of whom no longer spoke to one another. It was no wonder so many of the doctors were taking to drink and other dalliances. Thus, in more ways than one, the hospital had become a hotbed of seething turmoil. As a direct result of all this pressure, the wife of one of the doctors became a chronic kleptomaniac. She began shoplifting in local stores, but when the owners realized she was married to a physician and couldn't possibly be short of funds, they were nice enough to keep tabs and bill her husband once a month.

Stories about the Mendoza fracas appeared in several newspapers, but when one of the home town papers planned to do a follow-up, Dr. Cowgill phoned the editors and warned them not to print that story. "Dr. Mendoza is going to win his case against the hospital," he warned. A prophecy which eventually came to pass, incredibly enough.

About this same time, Dr. Cowgill intimidated a woman patient who had filed a complaint against both him and Dr. Mendoza. In this case, Mendoza's offense had been tantamount to a kidnapping. He put this woman in the intensive care unit, telling her that she'd had a heart attack when, in reality, there was nothing seriously wrong with her except minor indigestion. He kept her in the intensive care unit for about ten days, giving her the false impression that she was dangerously ill and, not incidentally, running up an enormous bill for her to pay.

When Dr. Cowgill heard about her official complaint, he telephoned the woman and threatened her abusively, warning her how sorry she would be if she dared go through with her complaint. His manner was so intimidating that the woman panicked, fearing he might actually do her some bodily harm if she carried out her complaint.

"What're you trying to do, ruin me?" he thundered on the phone. "I've had a sterling reputation in this town for many years!" By his own admission, he seemed to imply that the "sterling" part of his reputation was more tarnish than silver. You'd think he would be the first to know it was time to put himself out to pasture. But, like septuagenarian Supreme Court justices, doctors are a breed apart: they never know when it is time to climb down off their pedestal.

When the patient told me how Cowgill had threatened her, I contacted my friend at MSB, Dave Callisher. He phoned Dr. Cowgill and told him to cool it. "In case you've forgotten, Dr. Cowgill," Callisher told him, "you're in business to serve your patients, not to scare the hell out of them. Right now I'd say you people are having enough problems without your adding a charge of criminal harassment to the books." That did it: Dr. Cowgill softened his tactics and even apologized to the frightened patient.

When I saw, and mostly heard via the grapevine, what was brewing and stewing inside that hospital, I feared for anyone who happened to be a patient during those months. I was told by more than one of the nurses that the doctors were going berserk as a result of the added pressures of this feud. Many of them were over-prescribing drugs for themselves, and others were taking crazy risks by engaging in sexual trysts right on the premises. It was at this time that one of the staff doctors walked into the X-ray room and caught another doctor on the X-ray table atop a willing and euphoric-looking nurse.

"Oops, sorry, old pal," he scoffed. Then he softly closed the door and spread the story all over the hospital within half an hour. Even so, there *is* a limit to how willing these doctors will be to "inform" on one another. In most cases, each of them knows far too much about the others even to risk spreading nasty rumors. And because none of them have a clean enough record to be able to blow the whistle on anyone else, a conspiracy of silence was maintained among the staff; this unspoken bond existed between as many enemies as friends. They all kept tabs on one another for just this purpose, as if to say, "If you expose my crimes, I'll expose yours." I'm sure the same sort of "blood-brother pacts" are used to keep one Mafia member from killing another.

This is hardly the sort of "fraternal camaraderie" one expects from the most prestigious physicians in town. Neither does it promote the feeling of trust and reassurance one seeks when being admitted to a major hospital.

As for Dr. Mendoza's many offenses, despite his countersuit and all the support he received from the staff, none of those offenses were minor.

One of Mendoza's patients, an elderly man who was originally admitted for a routine checkup, was kept in the hospital for over sixty days. Actually, there was nothing wrong with him, but Mendoza had an all-encompassing diagnosis for such patients: "...an undetermined ailment." And earning his high fees, Mendoza would personally see to it that this ailment would go "undetermined" as long as possible. On his medical records, Mendoza would also add, "Patient complaining of nausea, stomach gas, with possible surgery indicated at a later date...." and a lot more of the same technical-sounding gibberish. Meanwhile, it was also Mendoza's policy to keep these patients so tranquilized with drugs that they rarely even observed the passing of the days and weeks.

One would think any reasonably alert and caring adult would want to know what's taking the doctors so long to find out what's wrong with them; perhaps they might even ask, "Why don't you stick me on the table and cut me open, or cut me free?" But it must be remembered that so many people in the area were provincial and unsophisticated; many never once ventured outside of the county. It wasn't in their nature to be suspicious or even question the decisions of these "experts." In short, they were simple, trusting souls, and that was a trait which doctors like Mendoza preyed upon.

When Dr. Mendoza finally released the elderly patient mentioned above, he sent the state medical welfare agency a bill for eighty thousand dollars, but the agency refused to pay more than twenty thousand dollars. This was another strategy Dr. Mendoza used, especially when dealing with state and federal medical aid programs. He would deliberately overbill because he maintained that he'd end up with a lot more than if he'd been accurate in his billing at the start.

During one of the many diagnostic procedures which Mendoza performed unnecessarily, he punctured the patient's intestines and the patient later died. Once again, no action was taken by the heirs, and a lid was kept on the whole affair.

Another doctor who worked at the same hospital, Dr. Todd Miramonte, clearly vied with Mendoza for the title "King of the Quacks." It was Dr. Miramonte who kept a woman patient in the hospital for two months, after diagnosing her condition as epilepsy, and treating her accordingly. After two months, the patient's sister called me and said her sister seemed to be getting worse every day, adding, "Mrs. Carroll, I'm afraid her doctor has misdiagnosed her case. How do we get her out of there?"

I did some research and discovered that any patient has the right to fire the doctor and obtain a release from the hospital. Admittedly, having heard of Miramonte's temper, I felt he'd probably put a voodoo curse on the woman before letting her leave. Nevertheless, we had the law on our side, so I drew up all the necessary documentation and took it to the patient.

When Miramonte realized he was actually about to lose a patient before he'd had time to bill her, he was infuriated.

"That woman is *my* patient!" he screamed at us. "How dare you try to take her out of here?"

But the patient waved her official papers in his face and said, "These are my legal rights, and this is Mrs. Paula Carroll. I suppose you've heard of her?"

Miramonte glowered at me and said nothing, though I'm sure he had recognized me on sight.

"Well, Mrs. Carroll is here to take me out of here, no matter what you say or do." Then she looked at me. "Isn't that right, Mrs. Carroll?"

Again Miramonte stared at me, and this time the expression on his face was so devilish, it was all I could do to muster up enough courage to smile bravely. "Yes, that's why I'm here," I said. Then I handed the documents to Miramonte. "It's all there, Doctor, in black and white."

When he read the papers, I'm sure he paid special attention to the word "misdiagnosed." In any case, he gave us no further problems. He signed her release and the patient was taken to Bay City Medical Center.

Here, they soon discovered that this woman did not have epilepsy, but was suffering from a brain tumor. For two months Miramonte had been treating her for a disease she didn't have while, all that time, her real condition was getting worse. Fortunately, they got to her in time. After surgery, they found that the tumor was benign. Still, this was another patient who chose not to sue her original doctor for malpractice. Like so many others, she wanted nothing more to do with the man who had almost been responsible for her death.

Meanwhile, Dr. Miramonte continued his good works. He prescribed an antibiotic over the phone for an eleven-year-old boy who had meningitis. The boy later died. This case was also covered up by the medical group. Miramonte also diagnosed a serious pancreas infection as the flu. When the patient's wife complained that her husband wasn't getting any better, Miramonte countered with, "Well, he's not getting any worse, either." That was about as cheerful as this doctor got when dispensing tender loving care. A week later this patient was taken up to a medical facility in Bay City. The doctors there said that if his condition had continued untreated for another five days, he would have died.

Another tragic case involved a patient by the name of Hiram Schultz who had been ill with undiagnosed lung cancer for six months. During that period, Dr. Miramonte had been treating him for bronchitis, prescribing various medications for that disease. Mr. Schultz kept telling Miramonte that he knew he was seriously sick.

"Don't be such a hypochondriac," Miramonte upbraided him. "All you have is a touch of bronchitis, so don't make such a big thing of it."

"But I'm coughing and wheezing, Doctor, can't you hear the wheezing in me? I can."

"Oh well," Miramonte scoffed, "nobody's perfect."

This went on and on while Mr. Schultz grew sicker and sicker. Finally, he confronted Miramonte and said, "Look, Doctor, I'm going up to Bay City. I want a second opinion."

When Miramonte knew that's what he was about to do, he called Mr. Schultz into his office, asking him to bring all his prescribed medication with him. Schultz complied. Dr. Miramonte looked at the bottles of pills and said, "I'm going to take you off all these pills at once. I'm convinced they're not helping you." Then Miramonte threw those pills down the garbage chute: he didn't want anyone to find out that he'd been treating this patient for a disease he didn't have.

When Schultz got to Bay City, within just a few hours they had him diagnosed as having inoperable lung cancer. After all those months, during which time Dr. Miramonte had obviously misread the original X-rays, he had continued to treat this cancer patient for bronchitis. Fortunately, Schultz had the presence of mind to go for the second opinion in time to learn he had a slow-growing cancer, which left him from one to three years to live. Had he remained under the care of Dr. Miramonte, his future would have been cut a lot shorter.

While it's appalling to remember that doctors like Miramonte, Mendoza, and their fellow-bunglers, Kearny, Post, Robins, Butler, et al., are still being allowed to practice it might seem even more horrifying to know what can happen to a doctor who tries to fight the system.

Such was the case of a young maverick by the name of Barry Tashlin. Dr. Tashlin, considered to be a genius by some of his colleagues, suffered under the delusion that he could change and improve the network of chicanery and greed that permeated the medical scene. He refused to join the professional organization and made it clear he didn't want to be involved with the game-playing tactics of the brotherhood.

Initially, the majority of his peers found subtle ways to tell him, "Don't get out of line." Ultimately, they weren't subtle at all. Dr. Tashlin, as it turned out, was not emotionally equipped to withstand the pressures that were exerted against him at the hospital. His inability to get along with other members of the medical profession, whom he criticized for a "country club" mentality and a materialistic drive, only added to the conflict and his pressures.

As a professional courtesy to the other doctors when they were on vacation he would see their post-op patients. However, those same doctors would refuse to reciprocate for him when he needed similar assistance. He was stripped of his staff privileges at the hospital where he performed surgery even though "he had never harmed anyone" and "no one ever accused him of malpractice."

After a few months, Dr. Tashlin began to show signs of the strain he was under. He became neurotic and unstable, and attempted to burn down the family home. Now, with a felony police charge against him, he was stripped of his license by the state.

One night, three months later, Barry Tashlin went home to his lonely apartment and was never seen alive again. He laid dead in his apartment for nearly a week before his body was found. The cause of death was never made clear. No toxocological tests were done because his body was too badly decomposed, and because foul play wasn't suspected.

In a newspaper account of his death, a psychiatrist contended that Tashlin was "hounded to death" by a medical-legal system intent upon punishing him for "delinquent" behavior rather than viewing him as physically ill.

Thus, the example was set for other ambitious young doctors who might want to step out of line.

Steve and I had been following the Tashlin case very closely. Because many of the nurses involved were loyal friends, I heard about the treatment this young man had endured from first-hand sources.

"This tragedy proves you can't be both a maverick and a doctor if you want to survive," Steve said after we read about Tashlin's death.

"That's very true," I said. Then, in an effort to cheer us both up, I added: "To get away with that, you have to be a consumer advocate. I mean, I'm not a doctor, so they can't 'get' to me the way they can persecute their own. They certainly can't put me through one of their 'impaired physician programs.' And I've already been through their 'impaired patient program' for years, so what more can they do to me?''

Chapter Twenty-three

*M*eanwhile, back at the hospital, where the feud still raged, those continuing warring factions were having other repercussions. One doctor dreamed up his own way to create a more stress-free environment, but it was a solution that backfired. He set up practice in another community. I guess he saw this as a surefire way to bail out if and when the medical pressure cooker finally blew its top.

But the high-handed tactics he got away with elsewhere did not endear him to that little town. When he tried to take charge and revamp the whole medical process there, they ousted him from the system. It had reached the point where people were refusing to go to the hospital because of his underhanded procedures. After only a few months, fearing their little hospital might go bankrupt, the administrators refused to let this doctor practice. They showed him the highway out of town, and strongly suggested that he didn't try for a return engagement.

I could well imagine his humiliation, to be thrown out of a two-by-four village like that. Unfortunately, not all of the offending doctors were given their just desserts in this fashion, not even those doctors who were known to be working in "diminished capacity." Instead of punishment, these men were given special treatment which would seem more appropriate for child prodigies.

I'm talking here about the alarming number of physicians and surgeons who were habitual alcoholics or drug addicts. There were occasions during which surgery had to be cancelled because the surgeon's pick-me-up booze intake hadn't steadied his hands sufficiently for him to operate.

One doctor, who had been up for a professorship in another town, was kicked out of a prestigious hospital because of his heavy drug problem. He came to town because, as he put it, "The word is that you don't have to *be* good to *look* good here."

But after only a year of practice, he started prescribing heavy doses of Demerol for himself, so he was in trouble again. He was so hooked on this narcotic, even his own nurse knew better than to talk to him before ten in the morning, as it was then that he had his first shot for the day.

Because of his addiction, many surgeries had to be cancelled, though not enough, unfortunately. One of his patients died when this doctor insisted on performing during a drugged stupor, and another young patient was left with permanent brain damage, a hopeful fifteen-year-old girl who would have had everything to live for, had it not been for her encounter with one doctor's diminished capacity. After the death of the other patient, it was reported that this doctor gave himself another shot of Demerol, then went into the records room. There he worked the medical records over, wanting to make sure the report would absolve him of any wrongdoing. In this regard, he had help. Within a period of twenty-four hours, five different changes were made on those records, contributed as a joint effort from all the principal physicians involved in the foul-up.

That's when the state moved in to chastise the addicted doctor. It must be noted, however, that when an alcoholic or drug-addicted doctor is "relieved" of his duties, what happens does, quite literally, come under the heading of "relief" rather than discipline. Once again, the aforementioned "impaired physician program" becomes a gentle rescue for these addicts. In this case, the offending doctor travels to Bay City once a week for drug therapy and counseling, but naturally, he is still being permitted to practice. The objective here is to show compassion and understanding to this poor addict, but certainly no one would be so cruel as to cut off his income.

Still another dope-ridden doctor, this one an anesthesiologist who was held responsible for two deaths during surgery, was known to do his billing while the patients were being operated on. He would "put them under," and then, instead of watching their vital signs closely, he would turn his back and do his paperwork. The nurses complained about this repeatedly. But not until two patients died as a result of anesthesia problems was this doctor "reassigned" long enough to be put through his own impaired physician program.

On the other hand, when a nurse without the right connections was recently accused of taking drugs on the job, she was fired without notice and arrested. No counseling, no therapy. To me, this double standard didn't make any sense, knowing that any doctor guilty of the same offense was treated so gently. Why fire a nurse and let the doctor go on practicing at his doped-up worst, when it's certain that he is in a position to do much more damage than she is?

However, this same treatment doesn't seem to apply when the offending nurse happens to have a husband on the hospital staff. I'm referring to the wife of Dr. Talbert—she is a court-declared drug addict. She has actually been arrested and jailed on drug charges. Nevertheless, she was welcomed back at the hospital with open arms as soon as her husband bailed her out.

When this case came to the attention of the state, they discovered that Dr. Talbert had actually been injecting his wife with morphine, and that he had also been giving her other hard drugs such as cocaine and Demerol for a period of two years before any action was taken. Finally, Dr. Talbert was arrested, for now there was no evading the issue: this man was a pusher and thus guilty of a felony.

But once again the double standard came to his rescue, and Talbert only got five year's probation, and was still free to practice. In other cases, some average citizen only had to be caught with a marijuana joint on him to end up serving a year's time on a road gang. Not so with these sacred cows.

Whenever I discuss this issue with my MSB friend, Dave Callisher, he lets me know how emphatically he agrees with my views. "Doctors who are heavily addicted to drugs or alcohol aren't 'impaired physicians.' These men are lushes or junkies, and whoever tries to see them as anything else needs more therapy than they do. These men are responsible for people's lives, so they should be given even more careful monitoring than normal street junkies, who can only harm themselves. Instead, they are humored, patronized, counseled, and coddled, then they're permitted to go on doing their worst to their innocent patients."

Another doctor, Dr. Maurice Pendergast, was all too obviously not cut out for his job. His offense occurred while he was performing a simple tonsillectomy in his office. The patient was a seven-year-old boy named Jonathan. The boy's mother sat waiting in the doctor's reception room for an interminable length of time.

Finally, the doctor came out and said, "I'm sorry, Mrs. Morrison, I'm afraid we ran into a little problem with Jonathan."

"What does that mean?"

"He died."

The poor woman gaped at him, too stunned to make a sound for a moment. "What are you talking about? I just brought him here to have his tonsils out."

"Yes, I know," Pendergast said with a little sigh. "It was one of those freak accidents that happen sometimes, when nobody's to blame. Of course, I don't have to tell you there's a certain element of risk during any surgical procedure."

Then Mrs. Morrison grew too hysterical to question him further. Despite this horror, she was another victim who refused to sign a complaint. And because the "Brotherhood" rallied around Pendergast with their support, it was never revealed exactly how he had killed that poor child. Of course, he and his nurse were alone in his treatment room at the time, so perhaps *she* could have made the fatal mistake. It's rare that the people present during these crimes will serve as witnesses; it's more likely they're accessories. Consequently, there is no limit to what these men can get away with.

But in the case of Dr. Pendergast, he had a lot of help from his peers. They had reason to know what a bungler he was. There was no way they would let this scandal leak to the public, so they figured their only alternative was to get this man into another branch of medicine, preferably where he didn't have such ready access to lethal weapons.

They had a special meeting and asked Pendergast what he would most like to do in the field of medicine—other than surgery, of course. He replied that he had always wanted to be an endocrinologist. Figuring he couldn't do much harm in this field, they sent him to a medical school in the midwest to receive training that got him out of their hair and sight for two years.

Once again, an "impaired"—and in this case, homicidal—physician was being rewarded instead of punished. If Dr. Pendergast hadn't killed that little boy, he might never have been given this opportunity. As I see it, the only service to the community this provided was getting this misfit out of surgery.

As for the little boy's mother, she had just lost her husband a few months earlier, so this double trauma left her too shaken up to take any action. In time of grief, many people are so immobilized by their own shock and depression, they can't see beyond the present.

When I urged Mrs. Morrison not to let them get away with this, she said something which so many others have said in the past when facing such a crisis. "Why bother, when it won't bring him back?"

She had a point there, of course, but if more people made these horrors known to the public, their action might give others the courage to launch their own protest in the future, and protect future unsuspecting and innocent patients.

While all this was going on, my former surgical assailant, Dr. Kearny, was at it again. He removed a perfectly healthy breast, certain it was cancerous. That's typical of the Kearny method of diagnosis. "I think maybe it's cancerous," he'll say, and because he's still a firm believer in that old adage "better sorry than safe," he wouldn't hesitate to start carving. If only that man's mind were half as sharp as his surgical tools.

Although the woman in this case is utterly devastated, and complains about this foul-up all over town, she, too, has refused to take any action. In her case, I had done all the necessary documentation and had even presented it to the state, but without her support, there is no case.

Kearny is also famous for *not* performing operations which any intern could have told him were necessary. The case I'm thinking of involved another woman cancer patient. She had a breast lump for over a year, but all Kearny said was, "Let's just wait and watch it."

He watched it until it became so bad, he finally performed the surgery. By then the cancer had spread throughout her body. As you'll recall, Kearny is the same amateur who fails to do complete cancer surgery when total excision is possible. He also refrains from telling people that he has found cancer during surgery.

When Kearny wasn't cutting off the wrong breast, or failing to remove the right one, he committed the same grisly blunders on the lower extremities. In short, he gravitated from breasts to legs, wielding the same indiscriminate carving knife. The worst example of such an offense was a collaboration between Kearny and his pal, Dr. Robins.

The patient was a man with a badly ulcerated leg. Kearny, who never wastes much time on indecision, said to Dr. Robins, "I think a fast amputation is indicated here." But this time Kearny cut off the wrong leg—the healthy one.

The patient and his family filed a big lawsuit against Kearny, who might well have said to these people, "You'll have to wait your turn, with all the others ahead of you."

With so many suits pending against this man, you would think the AMA would finally step in and prevent him from doing any more surgery. But that doesn't happen. All they will admit is that some of the doctors are dangerous. They never stipulate exactly which doctors they're talking about; they seem content to sit back and let the uninformed public play pot-luck with their lives. In most cases, the patient will never know when he's been unlucky enough to choose a dangerous doctor until the bad news shows up in his X-rays. By then it's too late.

Dr. Kearny is not improving with age; it's doubtful he'll be getting any more proficient. Most of his recent experience involves surgical blunders. As he's got that down so perfectly by now, one wonders how

163

he can perform any other way except incompetently? Old habits like these die hard.

Yet, despite Kearny's bloody trail of surgical victims, I would have to say that the now-legendary Dr. Albert Mendoza beat his record. Mendoza is a comparatively young man, so he cannot blame his blunders on decrepitude.

One of Mendoza's bungled cases involved a woman with a stomach ulcer, though Mendoza insisted on diagnosing her condition as cancer. Mendoza sent the patient to surgery and indicated to Dr. Post exactly which part of her cancerous stomach he wanted removed. That was Mendoza's second mistake. First, the wrong diagnosis, now the wrong part of the stomach. Even if they had known about the woman's ulcer, by following Mendoza's instructions, Post's surgical directions wouldn't have taken him anywhere near it.

The result: Post and his assistants removed the healthy part of the woman's stomach. Then everybody panicked. There was no way they could have known their mistake until *after* the cutting. One look and Dr. Post phoned Mendoza and said, "You indicated the wrong part of the stomach. I took out the healthy part."

"Then you might as well take it all out," Mendoza told him, referring to the stomach, of course.

"If I do that, she'll die," said Post.

"She's terminal anyway," said Mendoza.

Still believing Mendoza's original diagnosis, that this patient had terminal stomach cancer, Dr. Post started complete removal, then changed his mind and attempted a crude patch-up job. Later, they told the family the patient had begun hemorrhaging on the operating table. Following my advice, they got her to a Bay City hospital where a surgeon attempted to rebuild her stomach, to no avail. The patient died.

"I've never seen a worse case of butchery," the Bay City surgeon said, agreeing to testify when the case went to the state.

The sad and final commentary on this case was that the patient was originally suffering from such a mild ulcer, it could probably have been treated with medication.

Another horror story involved an obstetrician by the name of Carl Swanson. At the time of this atrocity, Swanson was "on report" for having performed far too many Caesarean sections. On the day in question, one of his patients was about to give birth. Swanson, who had privileges at two hospitals, was dividing his activities between both hospitals. That way, he probably figured, it wouldn't be noticed that he was performing too many of these operations at any one hospital. In

164

other words, instead of curbing his crimes, he was simply hiding them better.

That day Swanson happened to be on duty at one of these hospitals when the obstetrics nurse phoned from the other hospital and said, "Your patient, Mrs. Riley, is ready to deliver, Doctor. Please come over here immediately."

"You tell the patient to get in her car and drive over here," he ordered the nurse. "I'm too busy to be driving clear across town right now." I learned later that he was also having a bitter feud with the staff at the other hospital that week, so he was not about to cooperate with any requests coming from that source. The patient's needs, once again, were incidental.

The obstetrics nurse tried to convince Swanson that their patient was too close to delivering at this point; the danger of moving her could prove to be very risky.

"Look, you either get that patient over here at once," said Swanson, "or it'll be your job!"

The nurse did as Swanson ordered. She and the patient's husband, who had been waiting in the hall, went to the gurney and together walked Mrs. Riley out to the family car. Mr. Riley got behind the wheel, after they tried to get the agonized patient comfortable in the seat next to him. Then they drove across town to where Swanson was waiting.

But by that time, the patient had developed so many additional complications that Dr. Swanson had to do another Caesarean section. As a result, the baby was born dead, and for awhile, it appeared they might also lose the mother, though the crisis passed and she survived.

In this case, a doctor and two of the nurses on duty that day made a point of documenting exactly what happened. They brought their report to me and agreed this was a case that should definitely be challenged in court. They asked me to talk to the woman's mother who, as it turned out, happened to be an old friend of mine. Acting as a kind of family counselor and go-between, I spoke to her and told her what had happened. By then, Mr. and Mrs. Riley had questioned why Swanson hadn't agreed to deliver the baby much earlier, at the other hospital. So at least they were suspicious. But until they saw this report, they had no idea of all the facts in the case.

Mr. Riley was infuriated. "How the hell can they get away with something like that?" he demanded. "If it wasn't for Swanson, our baby would be alive."

"I agree," I told him. "It's more than just criminal negligence. At the very least, he could be charged with involuntary manslaughter. But all I can do is present you with the facts. It's up to you people to take this through the courts. If you don't, Swanson will not only get away with what he's done to you, he'll be free to go on doing it to other people."

They agreed to think it over and get back to me.

But that was several months ago, and I've heard nothing further from them. When I view such public apathy and think of all the crimes that go unpunished while the perpetrators aren't even penalized for their misdeeds, much less stripped of their licenses, it almost gets me discouraged. But it also makes me more determined in my efforts to alert the public. Of course, I'm not about to get angry enough for all of us. No, it's up to the rest of you out there to stand up and say, "We've had enough of these medical atrocities, and we're not going to take it any more...!"

Just think what a crowd it would make if enough of you stood up at once and voiced your righteous wrath. And who knows, if you work at it hard enough, it may even get to be a majority.

Chapter Twenty-four

*D*uring the course of CMQ's continued investigation into various medical atrocities, I learned of still another unethical practice that was all the rage at some hospitals. I got this inside information from several friendly nurses who, as it turned out, became my favorite hotline contacts to the hushed-up scandals among the doctors.

It seems that some doctors have the habit of hanging around the emergency room entrance to the hospital, simply because that's where all the money is. This is equally true of prestigious surgeons, internists, residents, and anesthesiologists. These men are like ambulance chasers in reverse. Wherever they happen to be on duty in the hospital, they listen for the sound of approaching sirens. When the sirens stop, that's their cue to run down to the emergency room admitting entrance, where the patients must settle for whichever doctors are on hand. In these crisis situations, especially cases involving accidents and trauma, the doctor can run every test in the book, then claim it's an emergency, so he's perfectly justified. In this way they can tally up a staggering amount of extra fees in one night.

But now and then, due to the heavy amount of pending malpractice cases, the greed of these doctors is sometimes overshadowed by their paranoia. As a case in point, when the daughter of an attorney recently had an accident and broke her leg, no doctor would agree to treat her. The simple fact that this patient's father was a lawyer made them afraid to go near her. When I heard about this, I discovered it was a known fact that some doctors are reluctant to treat an attorney or anyone related to an attorney.

However, not all the shocking cases of medical abuse occur in hospitals. A mental facility in a nearby town has also been the victim of this trend. This is a private institution, though it does take medical welfare patients. Not long after our group was formed, we began to receive constant complaints of criminal neglect and sexual abuse being doled out to the inmates by the staff here. After I collected all the necessary documentation on this facility, there were over twenty different citations written up against them. Young women patients were repeatedly beaten up by the staff if they refused to have sex. A subsequent state inspection revealed mold, filth, inedible food, live and exposed electric wires, parts of the ceiling falling down, no towels, and dirty linens.

The lid of secrecy was finally lifted one day when a delicate but attractive woman patient phoned her sister and in so many words said, ''Please send for the police so I can get away from this place.'' The state has opened an investigation, but one wonders why it takes so long when human suffering is needlessly taking place.

One of the most monstrous cases of neglect I've ever investigated was a matter of one family member mistreating another, though it was far more shocking than any typical battered-wife syndrome. And in this case, the negligence of the attending physician did nothing to alleviate the crisis.

The patient was a frail woman whose name was Marie Jameson. She has had a crippling disease for over nine years, and weighs less than eighty pounds. It wasn't until a social worker visited the Jameson house and saw the appalling conditions there that she notified MSB, who promptly urged her to contact me. Whereupon MSB sent in two investigators, inviting me to sit in on the meeting. Never had I heard such a revolting report of neglect and human cruelty.

This woman's husband has kept her imprisoned in her own home, forcing her to subsist in the filthiest conditions imaginable. She lays around in her excrement, unwashed and unattended. Unable to use the bathtub, the wife is bathed in an old horse trough in cold, dirty water. And because he never changes the water, it is full of slime and mold. The woman's own uncle also lives in this house, but he is terrified of his niece's sadistic husband.

During MSB's investigation, they tried to enlist the aid of several social agencies but because of bureaucratic red tape they were unable to take any action. In the course of nine years her only ''treatment'' has been an occasional delousing by her private physician, Dr. Paul Davidson. Certainly the doctor had to be aware of this woman's deteriorating condition over such a long period. Yet, he did only what Mr. Jameson asked him to do: he deloused a patient who was clearly in danger of dying from criminal neglect.

Upon learning how Davidson had actually contributed to this woman's neglect, MSB criticized him severely for not reporting her condition at once. It was even more incredible that, in rebuttal, Dr. Davidson wrote a letter to MSB, with copies to various other health agencies, and actually admitted, verbatim, that "...in my opinion, this man Jameson had devised this scheme to kill his wife...."

My MSB cohort, Dave Callisher, made a point of sending me a copy of this letter. Like Dave, I was amazed that Davidson would be foolish enough to admit his suspicions when it was also just as clear that he had never reported them to the authorities. Because Davidson knew about Marie's condition all those years and felt Jameson planned to kill his wife, he was, in fact, a consenting participant.

If Davidson had such fears all those years, you would think that out of normal curiosity he would want to follow up on it. He should have wondered why any woman would need to be deloused twice a month, and how was the husband involved, and what was going on at home. He should have reported these observations to the police at once. Instead, Davidson let it go on for nine years, and was then stupid enough to admit in writing how long he had been suspicious.

Finally, a social service agency stepped in and informed Marie Jameson it was her right to be moved to a convalescent home. But when I pursued this, they told me she had flatly refused this suggestion. I told them that was obviously because she was afraid to disobey her husband. I then reminded them there *were* alternatives: the court could go in and force that man to obtain the proper care for his wife.

Unfortunately, one agency keeps passing the buck to the next. As a result, Marie Jameson is still living in that daily nightmare, ill and imprisoned by her brute of a husband. Perhaps it won't be until she dies that the proper authorities will step in and prove the accuracy of Dr. Davidson's suspicions, that this woman's husband had, in truth, devised a surefire scheme to kill his wife.

In time, I forced myself to turn away from such heartbreaking frustrations by concentrating on the cases I *could* do something about, such as the woman who came to me after having a badly bungled hysterectomy. At first, Rosalind Ayres was too embarrassed to tell me her problem. But finally I got her to relax, and she told me a story I had heard before. I later learned that this time it involved a lady gynecologist, a Dr. Brolin. Once again, it appeared she had nicked a patient's bladder during surgery.

"I've had to resort to wearing Pampers, Mrs. Carroll," Mrs. Ayres told me. "In fact, I went through thirty-six of them in the last thirty-six hours." In time I was able to get her to another doctor. She had corrective surgery and fortunately did not need a urostomy, which would have entailed having a bladder bag attached to the leg. However, before this happened, Mrs. Ayres encountered another obstacle.

Before coming to me, she called a new 800 number that put her in touch with a centrally located service that now gives out the names of doctors in certain areas, whenever a patient calls seeking someone to consult for a second opinion. But apparently the person whose number she was given advised Mrs. Ayres to go back to her original doctor. "You should really be more civic-minded and support your local doctor," the man told her. "Why not give her a fair chance?"

Mrs. Ayres, feeling that she'd already given her doctor a chance to foul up once, was in no mood to ask for an encore. She reported this to me, then added, "After that phone call, he must have called Dr. Brolin and told her how I had asked for a second opinion behind her back. So she phoned me and was very abusive. She told me she was insulted to think I would dare seek a second opinion and try to ruin her reputation. Well, I just thought that was too much, so I said, "What are *you* angry about? I'm the one who has to wear Pampers at my age, not you!" Then I hung up. Now I still don't know what good it did for me to call that 800 number. The man I spoke to made me feel like a criminal, just because I wanted a second opinion."

I called the 800 number and asked to speak to the head of the service. She was good enough to give me the phone number they gave out whenever someone in the area called seeking a second opinion. When I wrote the number down, I recognized it at once. It was the number of a referral agency for doctors. When I told her what happened to Mrs. Ayres, she said it was the most outrageous incident she'd ever heard of.

"We've offered this service for three years, and we've never had anything like this happen. How very unprofessional!"

"Not in this area, I'm afraid," I said. "Here such medical collusion is par for the course. Now I'm wondering how long they've been doing this. There could have been a lot of other cases I wouldn't have heard about, and a lot of patients who should have sought a second opinion but were talked out of it."

"Yes, I see what you mean. That makes it even more outrageous. I'm going to call them right now and warn them that if they ever pull off such a stunt again, we'll strike their name and number from our records."

I warned her of the excuses she would get when she called the referral agency. When she called back a half hour later, she said, "You were right about the excuses, Mrs. Carroll. Incidentally, how many people work in that office?"

"One—a man named Douglas," I replied. "He works alone."

"I rather suspected as much. He stammered out his excuses, saying it must have been another of his workers who answered the phone. So I told him to give that 'other worker' a message for me: if anyone in that office ever tried that again, the agency would be stripped from our records, *and* reported to the appropriate state agencies."

As it happened, while Steve and I were out to dinner that evening, who should we see going out of the restaurant as we came in but Ed Douglas. He turned away from us without a word.

"I think he's had a bad day," I told Steve.

"And learned a lesson," he replied.

As time passed, it became more of a challenge to be exposed to all these tragedies without getting emotionally upset. And yet I knew that the only way I could really be of service to these people was to try and spare them my feelings; they were already experiencing enough adverse feelings of their own. In time, I learned to show them how much I cared without becoming overly maudlin or sentimental. What they needed was my help, not my pity. I now realized the sort of distance and objectivity most social workers must convey if they want to go on serving so many troubled people without losing control of their own emotions. It's quite a knack, learning how to be concerned and detached at the same time, but when it helps others, it's surprising how easy it is to pick up the habit.

In my case, when people knew of my own harrowing medical experiences, it could sometimes be helpful. But I did not make a point of discussing my background with them. It was their problems we concentrated on, not mine. So many of these people faced a life-threatening crisis; it really wouldn't help them if I were to say, "You think *your* life is up for grabs? Wait'll you hear how many times *I* was given up as a lost cause!" That sort of complaining would have little bearing on their present situation, which needed fast solutions in the present, not a pointless discussion of how much worse things were for me in the past.

Mostly I share my medical knowledge and experience with these people, not my agony. Indeed, though they may not know it, my being able to solve their problems keeps me from remembering how awful things used to be for me. In that way I feel it's an even trade.

Of course, when cancer patients come to me for guidance, I feel a special rapport with them. I remember one case in particular involving a woman by the name of Regina Tucker. She'd had a recent mastectomy, and in this case, it wasn't her doctors who had victimized her, it was the people who had sold and fitted her for a prosthesis. She was having enough problems adjusting to her surgery without the added discomfort of having to wear a badly fitted prosthesis, as it only intensified her pain.

When Mrs. Tucker said she had purchased the prosthesis at a local store, she and I drove there together. I told her she had the right to demand a refund. "I suggested that on the phone," she replied, "but they told me they never give refunds. It's against company policy."

"Well, I have news for them," I said. "That policy just lapsed, as of today."

When we arrived at the shop, I explained to the woman how badly Mrs. Tucker had been fitted. "How would you feel if you were in her position?" I asked the manager. "Here she's just learned she has cancer, has had a breast removed, and now, before she's even had time to adjust to the shock, you sell her a prosthesis that was obviously designed for another woman. You think she needs all that additional pain right now, and at these prices? I feel the least you can do is give her a full refund."

Of course, before I made this speech, I had already presented her with our card, identifying myself as a consumer advocate. The woman apologized profusely. And even while she kept repeating "it's against our policy," she was at the cash register, counting out the bills.

Later that week, Mrs. Tucker and I drove to the place where I had obtained my prosthesis, though it had taken me a lot of hit-and-miss tries to find it. There I had her fitted as she should have been at the start.

This is the sort of service I provide, and frankly, I derive a great deal of personal satisfaction in being able to right some of the wrongs for others that were done to me in the past. How I wish I'd had a place like CMQ to go to during the years when I was going around in circles, my mind a maze of doubts and unanswered questions.

Another case that inspired similar fast action involved a terminal lung cancer patient whose lung cancer was first misdiagnosed as TB and he was sent through the TB clinic for treatment. This was a patient by the name of Kyle Houston. After a long hospitalization, he had recently been sent home; though we knew he didn't have long to live, when we heard about the unique way he was victimized, we wasted no time in setting things right. At home, Houston and his wife paid three hundred dollars to have a hospital bed and other medical equipment delivered. Apparently nobody at the hospital had told him that all this equipment is available to cancer patients free of charge, through the auspices of the Cancer Society. To make matters worse, this family was so destitute, we had been helping them financially via our Emergency Loan Fund. They had spent their last three hundred dollars for a month's rent for equipment that should have gone to them free of charge, if the doctors had only told them about it.

When I heard about this, I called the firm where he had rented the

172

equipment and told the receptionist that she should have informed the patient he was eligible to get this equipment free of charge.

"Why would you do a thing like this?" I asked her on the phone. "These people are so destitute, they don't even have food in the house. Meanwhile, we'll be willing to pay the charges for pickup and sterilization. But please refund the money."

I guess I really rattled her cage, as I could tell she was less than delighted with my attitude. We went a few rounds on the phone, but I won and the Houstons got their money back. There are too many greedy people waiting to profit from the misery of others.

Only a few days later the public nurse who had been looking in on Kyle Houston phoned to tell me he had died in the night. "But you know something, Mrs. Carroll," she said, "speaking for the family, the best thing that happened out of all this was getting to meet you and learning about your group. Now that we know who and where you are, we're going to help spread the good word."

Before I even had time to mourn that poor man, I received a call from another cancer patient, and her complaint made me too angry to feel depressed. This was a sweet little lady by the name of Emily Hammond. She had cervical cancer, and at the time of her call, she was receiving radiation therapy.

"Mrs. Carroll, I don't know if it's because of the radiation or what," she said, "but suddenly I got very sick with diarrhea. Then I told my doctor about it, and he said, 'Oh, it's all in your head.' Now what do you think of that?"

"I think, among other things, that this doctor of yours has a poor sense of direction."

"Well, you know how Dr. Butler is," she said. "He's so temperamental and unpredictable."

Butler! I thought, remembering the trouble he had given me early in my illness. As I recalled, he had all the warmth and compassion of a cobra. To help Emily Hammond, I did some research on diarrhea, picked out several pamphlets on the subject and brought them to her. In no time at all, she was much improved.

During my visit to her bedside at home, she received phone calls from Dr. Butler, from her radiation therapist, and also from a nurse. Each of these people gave her different, though equally officious, orders, until the poor woman was almost in a state of panic. But it was her meek and submissive manner while speaking to her doctor that disturbed me the most. I could tell by her attitude that he was angry with her.

"I'm sorry, Doctor...I'm not mad at you. Please forgive me...."

I thought it was pitiful for her to be so humble and obsequious, when he should have done all the apologizing. Yet, recalling my own experience, I could well understand Mrs. Hammond's fear of offending these doctors, lest they refuse to treat her. When she hung up the phone that day, she smiled sweetly at me. "I always feel it's best if you don't upset them, you know? They're very sensitive people, and high-strung, too, like *prima donnas*. So I try my best to please them."

It wasn't easy, but on this subject I keep my opinions to myself. Mrs. Hammond was in her seventies, on Medicare, with very few alternatives, so what good would it do to tell her that these "prima donnas" didn't deserve to be coddled? Instead, they could all use a six-month crash course at the nearest charm school, with a special class in "how *not* to browbeat the sick and the elderly...."

Chapter Twenty-five

*N*o matter how many potential medical disasters we were able to prevent through the services of our group, "exceptional" incidents of fraud, conspiracy, and butchery were still brought to our attention much too late for us to do anything but help the victims file a complaint.

Take the case of Wilbur Sandford, a man in his sixties. He was admitted to the hospital with an ulcer of the esophagus, which isn't considered terribly serious, if you get the right treatment in time, and from the right doctors. But this patient was at the mercy of a woman doctor named Lee Derringer. Dr. Derringer was notable for having left her practice for a period of ten years to become a financier, with her husband, in New York. After filing bankruptcy, she was forced to return to her medical practice. Although she hadn't touched a scalpel in ten years, she said, "Oh, I can pick it up again in a jiffy. It's like riding a bike: you never forget."

But she proved herself wrong when Wilbur Sandford came to her, at a time when Derringer had only been back in the harness for three weeks. She was forced to take this patient back to surgery four times within one month just to repair her previous surgical mistakes. Each "repair" left Sandford in more critical condition. During the final surgery, Dr. Derringer inserted a balloon ring around the esophagus as a means of preventing excessive bleeding following a tracheotomy.

But this device was so ineptly placed, it cut into the tissue and the patient died of internal bleeding. I spoke to Sandford's brother, who signed the complaint to the state. Weeping, he told me he was in the room with his brother at the very last. "He was conscious and he knew something was wrong. He was clutching at his throat, trying to free himself from that thing that must have been strangling him. When I pointed this out to the doctor, she said I was mistaken, that my brother was just reacting to the heavy sedation, implying that he was delirious."

To confuse the issue, Sandford's death certificate, signed by Derringer, listed ten different possible causes of death and unwittingly outlined the surgical mistakes that had been made. Nevertheless, after conducting their investigation, MSB stated this was one of the most appalling cases of surgical bungling on record. While the case is pending, Dr. Derringer is still on duty at the hospital, determined to regain the same surgical flair she had before her ten-year hiatus as a failed financier. With that "hit and miss" philosophy, one wonders if she or her patients will ever come out ahead. First they'd have to come out of the anesthesia, and with Derringer at the helm, that, too, is doubtful.

Through the grapevine, I heard about Derringer's next gamble: she treated a woman for hemorrhoids. Her condition worsened, so she contacted me and I advised her to get a second opinion. Instead of hemorrhoids, the woman had rectal cancer. This case is also pending.

One of the most pathetic cases I've ever handled involved a twenty-three-year-old mother of three small children. This woman, whose name is Diana Bailey, is a paraplegic, confined to a wheelchair. She had a decubitus ulcer (a bedsore) at the base of her spine that was so deep, the muscle and bone could be seen. But because she was paralyzed from the waist down, Mrs. Bailey had no idea the sore was so advanced. Then her husband saw it and quickly got her to a doctor, who removed the unhealthy tissue. He tried to pull the tissue together, but the stitches kept tearing out. She endured that condition, off and on, for a year. It was so bad, it's a wonder it didn't become gangrenous. She finally changed doctors, and this time she ended up with the gruff and ill-natured Dr. Miramonte.

When she first went to Miramonte for treatment, she had a temperature of 103 and was so overwrought she began to cry. "What're you crying about?" Miramonte barked at her as she lay on his examination table, apparently unconcerned that the woman's husband and a social worker were also present. "I know what your trouble is," he went on. "You're lazy. Why don't you get off your butt instead of sitting around in a wheelchair all day?"

"Hey, now wait a minute...." Mr. Bailey burst out.

"Dr. Miramonte," said the social worker, "has it escaped your attention that this woman is a paraplegic? If you'd read her chart more carefully, I wouldn't have to tell you that...."

Miramonte glared at her. "Look, if I sat around reading charts all day, I'd never get anything done!"

When I heard this later, I thought: what a boon to all his patients that would be.

Finally, Miramonte admitted Mrs. Bailey to the hospital and attempted, without success, to debride her ulcer.

When his attempt was unsuccessful, he nonchalantly explained, "You'll just have to live with it."

It was at that point that Mrs. Bailey and her social worker came to me, and I directed them to a Bay City hospital. There, the doctors performed a skin graft and within three weeks, the ulcer was completely healed.

Now we come to the case of Dolores DeVega. Despite the fact that no less than five doctors had examined her, she had undiagnosed thyroid cancer for a period of ten months, from January, 1982, until October of the same year.

Her first doctor was unable to diagnose her ailment. He sent her to four other doctors and they were also unable to come up with a diagnosis. Mrs. DeVega felt she had reached the end of her rope. She kept going back every two or three weeks, and all they could tell her was something she already knew: "You've got a severe pain in the neck." They suggested she use a heating pad and pain pills.

That is precisely what she did: she began to self-treat her neck with heat and aspirin. One of the five doctors came up with a "theory" of what he thought her ailment might be. He said, "What you have *could* be gastric acid backing up from the stomach into the throat area." Not that he'd ever treated such an ailment before. Still, he even drew a diagram of this theory to show her how it might be happening. Meanwhile, Mrs. DeVega had an enormous lump at the side of her neck.

By then, it was October of 1982, and because even these bunglers could recognize a lump when they saw one, they finally performed a biopsy and found a tumor. But again they misdiagnosed and said the tumor was benign.

It wasn't until later, when I got Mrs. DeVega up to a Bay City hospital, that the correct diagnosis was made: she had what was believed to be the most virulent form of neck cancer.

This case wasn't brought to my attention until after she'd had the "benign" biopsy. The woman's husband called me at that time and said, "It's benign, but they want to do radiation."

I was able to get Mrs. DeVega an appointment up at Bay City hospital. When the doctors there reviewed the original X-rays that were taken in January, they all agreed that the tumor had been clearly visible way back then, and wondered why her doctors hadn't detected it at that time. If they had, they said her prognosis would have been excellent back in January. But now it was too late—she was terminal. There was nothing more to be done for her, except to send her back home to wait for death.

We became closely involved with another young woman and her husband because they were destitute, and because the woman, whose name was Anita Sanders, was suffering from an all-but-untreatable disease called aplastic anemia. This is similar to leukemia, though it is not a cancer. Because there is no known cure for it, it is harder to treat than leukemia.

One morning last August, I got a desperate phone call from Anita, who was in the hospital. She complained that the doctors had given her the wrong medication and it was throwing her into a nervous tailspin. She seemed frantic on the phone and pleaded with me to come visit her at the hospital.

"Now Anita, they've got you in isolation in the intensive care unit," I reminded her. "And it's only six in the morning, long before visiting hours. And we're not family, so I doubt they'd let us see you."

"Yes they will," she insisted, "because I'll tell them to!"

Despite the early hour, Steve and I got up and got dressed. We drove to the hospital and went directly to the intensive care unit. The doctor emerged from the room at that moment, and though he wore the usual surgical mask, I saw at once that this was the comparatively harmless Dr. Forbes. He also recognized me at once. "We'll be finished with the patient in a moment," he told us. "Then you can go in and see her."

While Steve and I waited, they gowned and masked us both. Then we went in and had a long, relaxed visit with Anita. It meant a lot to her to know there was someone close who really cared about her. She poured out all her frustrations, explained how they had given her the wrong medication due to some red tape or getting her chart switched with someone else's. Stories like these were all too familiar to me, since I had done my own time at this hospital. Anita told me she wanted to be transferred back to a hospital in her area where she felt she'd have a better chance to get well.

I called her doctor at this hospital, and he was so nasty on the phone, I wondered why she would want to return to him. "I am sick and tired of that woman and her case!" he shouted. "And I am tired of this patient's impossible demands!"

About two weeks later, Anita died. Because she and her husband had been in such dire straits, our group held a big fund-raising meeting to help her impoverished survivors, which included two small children.

Not long after Anita's funeral, another doctor mistakenly called in the wrong patient after presumably reading her alarming EKG. He ordered her to show up at the hospital's intensive care unit immediately, as she was dangerously ill. "You get here at once," he shouted over the phone, "or I'll send an ambulance for you!"

The patient, Mrs. Chatterson, later told me how amazed she was by this call. She had just been at the hospital for a routine physical, and before being released, they told her that her EKG had been perfectly normal. Nevertheless, she went to the hospital and spent six hours in the intensive care unit.

Finally, the doctor who had phoned her came in and stared at her in astonishment. "Who the hell are you and what are you doing here?" As it turned out, she didn't recognize him either, because he wasn't even her doctor. There's no telling what sort of an "attack," psychosomatic or otherwise, Mrs. Chatterson might have had during those hours while she waited to expire from cardiac arrest at any moment. Naturally, this experience gave her quite a fright, and an expensive one, too. Her bill, which was processed through the computer at the time of her admission, came to one thousand dollars. She filed a complaint, of course, and that, too, is "pending."

It's even more ominous to speculate about the fate of the woman whose "alarming" EKG this doctor had actually read. If she was that "dangerously ill," one wonders what that added delay did to her condition. Perhaps a close study of that week's obituaries might have answered this question.

During some of my recent research, I learned that criminal incompetence among doctors is not as unique as I thought. Neither are the disastrous results faced by patients who are at the mercy of such ineptitude.

I heard of a doctor who enjoys the dubious privilege of getting all the botched-up garbage created by other blundering doctors in the state. It then becomes his job to act as custodian for these patients until they die—a custodian of the doomed and the mangled. The original blunderers apparently trust this ghoul with their most irretrievable mistakes. One wonders what sort of explanation is given to the heirs of all this "human garbage," although knowing as much as I do about medical coverups, I'm sure the ultimate records will imply "death by natural causes."

Among doctors, it is still considered unethical to warn a patient that a doctor he intends to use is incompetent, even though such a warning might save that patient's life. In this way, the ethics of the medical profession are served, but the patient may die as witness to its power to successfully withhold vital information. If the patient does discover the

179

truth, he is discredited at all costs and, in a sense, he suddenly becomes the criminal, the guilty one. In order to find a malpractice attorney, any person living in a small town must go to a larger city, which may often be so far away that the whole idea is impractical. Moreover, malpractice lawyers are often unwilling to practice in small towns in view of the small settlements that are usually involved.

So where does the justice come from? These cases are never judged purely on principle. Money, power, and reputation—these are the only determining factors, all adding up to greed on a very large scale, the kind of greed that seems to be contagious within the close-knit ranks of most doctors. One doctor sees a colleague earning enough to buy up half the real estate in town, so naturally he is envious and wants to play one-upsmanship, so he raises his fees and tries to see more patients per day than he can humanly handle. These doctors are no longer motivated primarily by a humanitarian concern for their patients. Their hunger to make a profit has taken top priority and therein lies the epidemic: greed in medicine.

It is disturbing to realize the power one profession continues to have over our lives. In our misguided endeavor to protect the elite of our society by our silent approval of their actions, we have only contributed to the crisis of disintegrating medical quality.

If you doubt this, consider this shocking information I recently received from two top state investigators. They told me about a very unique "workshop" now run by doctors, *for* doctors: a seminar dedicated to teaching them the fine art of remaining just this side of the law. In other words, how to stay in the "grey area" so the state won't prosecute them for medical welfare billing abuses. These seminars are now being conducted all over the state. Qualified experts in high finance have been engaged to teach the doctors how to get away with profitable billing abuses while avoiding the bothersome nuisance of getting caught.

This is not hearsay or gossip, mind you, for it has all been confirmed and the MSB is now investigating the problem. Even more disturbing, I'm told this has been going on for years and is a well-guarded secret. But in view of all our recently uncovered evidence, this is one secret society that will soon be forced up from the underground.

Of course, it is never an easy task to clearly define incompetence. Some states don't define it at all, and they also fail to actually pinpoint what is considered to be a disciplinary act. There seem to be no concrete clues or guidelines as to when a doctor should be penalized or investigated for incompetence. Yet the so-called malpractice crisis was caused only by the incompetence of doctors, nothing else. Statistics tell us that ninety percent of the malpractice suits are caused by ten percent of the doctors, and it is reasonable to believe that it is the hardcore incompetents who are causing most of the problems.

On the other hand, their policy of "confidentiality" remains the same: no names please, and no pointing the finger at any specific bungler. After all, that wouldn't be sporting.

Chapter Twenty-six

*A*fter we succeeded in filing our medical malpractice claim in the courts we were informed by the attorney that we had five years to proceed with legal action. It was believed that I could, very possibly, have a recurrence of my thyroid cancer because of Kearny's negligence. For this reason we were advised not to be hasty in a settlement of the claim. This five-year period would also give us ample time to find the best attorney for our case.

Approximately one year later we thought we had found the *right* attorney, but this proved to be a disappointing choice. Unfortunately, he was not as well-versed in the specialty of medical malpractice as we had first believed.

In December of 1982, the doctors discovered I had a recurrence of my thyroid cancer. This necessitated more tests and radioactive iodine treatments, and the possibility of additional surgery loomed once again.

I was determined that this setback would not interfere with my plans to help others. I continued to remain active in my organization's endeavors. Frankly, I had so many plans and ideas to nurture that I didn't have time to be sick.

Of course, we were gravely concerned over the status of my health and with this new development we again began our search for an attorney.

By February of 1983, we succeeded in finding the lawyer that I only wish we had found at the beginning of our legal challenge. I am certain everything, legally speaking, would have been far easier for us if we had met this attorney at the outset of our legal journey.

He had a strong moral code, he had principles, and his primary concerns were to challenge and change the system for the benefit of others.

Steve and I made several lengthy trips to his office to consult with him. After reviewing my medical records with his medical experts he agreed to take my case. By this time it was the end of February, 1983.

On the night of March 1, 1983, before our new attorney had had the chance to officially become our attorney of record, he telephoned us with some startling news. After reviewing our court filing papers, he realized that the documents had not been served to the defendants (the doctors and hospital). This *had* to be done within three years of the filing date. The deadline was two days away—March 3, 1983.

Of course, we had not realized that the papers hadn't been served. We had naturally assumed this had been done at the time of the filing.

Because of his great distance from us and the zero-hour deadline, our attorney told us by telephone how to hire a process server and get the papers served to the defendants.

There was a mad flurry of phone calls and paperwork. By four o'clock on March 3, 1983, we believed we had accomplished the impossible. All defendants had been served their notices.

However, there was one detail that we, as novices, didn't realize was left undone.

The process server brought the signed documents back *to us* and we failed to return them to the court *before* five o'clock on March 3, 1983. What we had not understood was that the papers not only had to be served, they had to be *returned* to the court to meet the deadline. By the time they were returned to the court it was *too late*.

The attorney suggested that we appeal but after reviewing similar cases that had failed in their attempts to win an appeal, it seemed futile. We would be arguing about something other than my original complaint and this could conceivably drag on for years.

Of course, I was disappointed. I believed, as did many fine professionals in the medical and legal professions, that I had been wronged and that I had the right to ask for an accounting.

But, rather than feeling defeated by this ironic stroke of misunderstanding and seeming bad luck, I eventually came to feel relief that this aspect of my challenge had ended.

The *only* reason I had sought relief through the filing of my suit was because I wanted to change the system. But I was already accomplishing that goal in a much greater capacity through my work with other people in trying to help them avoid the pitfalls I had encountered.

Chapter Twenty-seven

*B*y now it must be clear exactly why I am involved in this work. On occasion, I do miss some of the personal activities and social involvements I have had to give up. But at this point in my life, I am totally committed to CMQ and believe fully that this is the purpose of my life. So many of my past hobbies seem so trivial compared to what I'm doing now. This presents some difficulties when old friends approach me and suggest I join them in pursuits which I used to pursue; now I feel they are so superficial and downright silly. I guess my new attitude puts them off, but the fact is, my values have changed, and so have I.

I love the challenge of this work, and the chance to talk to new people and perhaps enlighten them in a way which can change their lives for the better. Among my rewards are some of the critically ill people who have learned to disregard the ugliness of their situation and see only the beauty that is possible while they still remain alive. The need to overcome such ugliness is the challenge. To overcome, not to surrender.

By directing my energies outward, and learning how much I care about others less fortunate than myself, I've been able to find and give a new kind of love, just by showing how much I care whenever I'm needed.

I am still committed to my efforts to change the old system. Speaking for the patients, I say that we are no longer going to remain passive spectators when it comes to the quality of our own health care. We will no longer be gullible enough to believe the medical profession when they promise us they will police their own members.

We must also realize that the obsolete system of licensing physicians has never protected the consumer. What disturbs me the most is that once a doctor has received a license, he is licensed for life. Moreover, he gets that license at a time in his life when he is functioning at his best; though he may never again function that expertly, that one license covers him for a multitude of sins for thirty or forty years. He is never under scrutiny again, regardless of what may happen to him, over the years—drug dependency, mental disorder, alcoholism. The license stays the same, even though the quality of his treatment may have gone progressively downhill.

Because the physician is never retested, this means he has been given a permanent license to kill. Think of the many medical changes and advances that have occurred since some doctor in his fifties or sixties was first issued his license. Unless he happens to be particularly resourceful or research-minded, he needn't feel obliged to learn anything more than he knew when he graduated. Even the plumber or the electrician receives more scrutiny under the state's licensing agency.

Today, the ever-present need is for more "patient education." For example, even now some people still choose their doctors by the most outmoded standards. If a doctor does a beautiful job sewing a few stitches, does that mean—as some patients assume—that he will be a genius in *any* medical situation? Not by any stretch of the imagination could you call that clear or deductive reasoning.

Neither does it follow that a surgeon who is brilliant at removing warts would be the best man to go to for radical cancer surgery. Regardless of how you may adore this man's smile, if you're still judging him by those old "wart" standards, you're in trouble. Yet some patients have only to see that decades-old diploma framed on the doctor's wall, and they willingly place their very lives in this man's hands. That is another defunct myth which we at CMQ hope to put to rest.

To begin to address the problems I have outlined, we medical consumers must assume more responsibility for our own health care. The concept of self-care puts more squarely on our shoulders the obligation to *listen* to our bodies before deciding on treatment. All response to sickness starts with the process of "listening" to the pain and the other signals your body sends to you. Don't be so eager to go to a doctor and let *him* tell you where it hurts. You know better than anyone where the pain is coming from, how long it has lasted. There's no need for you to wait for him to "draw assumptions," or lump you with scores of other patients in your general age bracket. Only you are responsible for the knowledge this man has of you. Too many of us are all too willing to put our fate in our doctor's hands when we go for treatment, but the process of regaining health must be a collaboration. Doctors are not psychic; they can't really know about our symptoms unless we talk to them, and in great detail.

In short, these men are not gods. They are fallible human beings who make mistakes. And until we impress on them that we are watching every move they make, they'll go on making more mistakes.

It is amazing how many people continue to make excuses for these so-called "men of honor." People point their finger at me and say, "You didn't die, Paula, you should be grateful!" Of course I'm grateful, for having the sense to get that second opinion in time to save my life. But certainly I feel no gratitude for those blundering doctors who left me in such a critical condition. That's like saying I should be grateful to a potential murderer because his gun misfired.

It has always been clear to me why these men fought me so hard: they knew I was getting close to the truth. If I wasn't, why would they have gone to so much trouble to discredit me? If, as they claimed, I had no reasons for my complaints, why did they overreact? Why didn't they simply ignore the "hysterical fool" they wanted others to think I was? It was their overreaction that convinced me there was a sound basis to all my accusations.

Now I have the satisfaction of knowing I did everything in my power to uncover the truth, and in doing so, I rattled—and I'm still rattling!—a lot of medical cages.

They will remember me now, the guilty ones. And now that I've launched my thriving consumer advocate group, several of them will never be the same because of their original conspiracy against me. Perhaps they didn't know it at the time, but they lit a powerful fuse when they started playing their tricks on me. Thanks to them, that fuse is still burning, brighter than ever.

I feel if I can alert even five percent of an inept doctor's patients, meaning one in twenty patients that the bungler sees, then perhaps it will be enough to stir up the others. If this happens, I will have achieved a resounding personal victory. And with this book serving as my one true and lasting forum, perhaps I will make the system a little better for those medical victims who may follow me in the future.

Epilogue

aula, you have zeroed right in on the heart of the problem,"
said the Executive Director of the Medical Standards Board,
when he learned of my library and my determination to provide medical
consumers with information that would enable them to make informed
choices regarding their medical and health care.

I had met with the director in his executive offices on several occasions.
In the Spring of 1983, he accepted my invitation to come to our area and
speak on issues concerning the medical consumer.

Addressing an audience of approximately 150 persons, including several doctors, he said, "The kindest thing I can say is that ten percent of
the physicians who are practicing today should not be practicing in a totally unconstrained environment."

Two days later, the newspapers carried the story of his talk. There was
an immediate outcry from the state medical association and other medical
groups. The president of the association fired off a letter to the Governor
of the state demanding that the director resign immediately and that he
apologize to the doctors and the public for his remarks. This demand was
absurd in light of the fact that the public—the medical consumers—must
know that ten percent of all doctors are incompetent to some degree.

Never once did this president attempt to find out what the director had
actually said. His actions were based solely on the news story and taken
out of context. It was an outrageous, hysterical demonstration of the
power of the medical profession against someone who would dare to
speak the truth. It was disturbing to witness the heavy-handed tactics
used by these professional associations to suppress the truth. What were
they afraid of? The director of the MSB was, most definitely, in a

position to know the facts. It was his agency's responsibility to license and discipline the state's physicians.

Following all the publicity generated by the talk, I received telephone calls from newspaper reporters and radio and television stations, asking for my comments on this disgraceful turn of events. For more than a month the sniping continued. I wrote a letter to the Governor attempting to explain that the director was very fair to both sides and that the whole matter had been taken out of context. But his powerful opponents were not going to let the director off the hook. They persisted with their demands until, finally, he resigned. Freedom of speech suffered a grave defeat and politics of the worst kind triumphed. I was deeply saddened when he called and told me that he would be leaving the agency as of June 1, 1983.

In spite of this temporary setback, our organization continued to grow and flourish. The public's interest in my endeavors rapidly increased. I continued to receive invitations to appear on television programs and radio talk shows. Numerous newspaper articles were published, and some of these were carried nationwide. Invitations to speak to various groups and organizations throughout the state increased. As a result of all this publicity, our organization received comments and requests for information from thousands of persons living in thirty-one states. In addition to serving as a consumer advocate, I have driven some patients to major medical centers in the state so they could receive the best medical care.

Even with the serious and somber issues that constantly confront me, there is always a story that gives rise to a chuckle or two. A woman called me who had been diagnosed by Dr. Forbes as having possible breast cancer. She explained to me that she did not want to go to Dr. Forbes or any of the other local doctors for the needed surgery and the post-op follow-up. She requested that I refer her to my doctor in Bay City. (Incidentally, she did not know about my experience with Dr. Forbes.) When she told Dr. Forbes that she was going to Paula Carroll's doctor in Bay City, ". . . he hit the ceiling." She said to me, "I can't understand why Forbes is so mad." I assured her not to worry about it for it was *his* problem.

I continue to learn more disturbing facts about both physician and hospital incompetence. Patients have shared their stories with me and asked me to assist them in filing complaints with the Medical Standards Board. From these numerous complaint filings we have begun to accumulate information, disturbing information, that reveals a pattern of physician incompetency that has been consistently ignored and unchallenged by the MSB.

To further validate my concerns, in 1982 the state's Auditor General's Office (AGO) conducted an extensive audit (performance review) on the MSB and I was one of the persons they interviewed. I related how the Board had failed to take appropriate action against dangerous doctors, some of whom the Board agreed were a menace. I shared with them my extensive documentation. When the report was released, many of MSB's deficiencies were brought to light.

In 1984, the AGO conducted a second audit. Released in 1985, this report declared that the problems raised in the 1982 report had not been corrected and additional serious deficiencies were outlined. This latest report carried the title: THE STATE'S DIVERSION PROGRAMS DO NOT ADEQUATELY PROTECT THE PUBLIC FROM HEALTH PROFESSIONALS WHO SUFFER FROM ALCOHOLISM OR DRUG ABUSE.

These shocking reports were not a surprise to me. *This* was the system I had tried to work within since 1977. I knew first-hand of the incompetence of the MSB. These disclosures only served to bear out the concerns I had felt for many years.

Over a period of several years I made countless long trips to meet with various MSB officials. I endeavored to understand the system, for it was, after all, the medical consumer's agency. Though its sole purpose was to represent the patient, the medical consumer, it had become the handservant of the medical associations.

Not only has this agency proven to be inept and ineffective, it is also insensitive to the tragedies that result because of its negligence. One MSB investigator said to me, "People are stupid...they're like a bunch of sheep. They deserve what they get."

I countered, "I take issue with that comment. The medical consumers are not allowed access to information that could protect them from incompetent, dangerous doctors. The profession and the state agencies dogmatically refuse to release even the minimal amount of data so we could be informed consumers. Your statement would only be correct if patients were allowed access to this information and then failed to act on it."

"That's true," he replied, nodding his head in agreement. "I have the feeling you're determined. In fact, I know you're tenacious, Paula."

"You're absolutely right. I'm going to make sure people are safe from the very doctors you and the state are protecting by concealing the facts from us."

How is this going to be accomplished?

A medical malpractice insurance executive once shared this thought with me: "Until the MSB is taken out of the hands of the politicians there will be no effective changes."

I quickly added, "There will be no effective changes until we, the medical consumers, demand them. Those of us who pay the bills must be considered and consulted in the decision-making process of how our health care system is operated and how our money is being spent. We want proof that the physician we choose and entrust with our lives is worthy of our trust."

Why do people hesitate to speak up? They are held hostage to their own fears and attitudes when they fail to challenge substandard medical care. Perhaps they want to believe that the medical profession is effectively policing its own members.

A short time ago, I met with a physician who was lamenting the high cost of medical malpractice insurance. I questioned, "Why don't you get rid of the bad doctors? Why do you put up with high-risk, incompetent doctors? By doing so you are driving up your own insurance rates."

"Paula, I can't," he answered candidly. "I've got skeletons in my closet, too. If I blow the whistle on a colleague he'll turn around and blow the whistle on me."

"Isn't that a tragedy," I replied. "But the tragedy falls mostly to the unsuspecting patients who believe you are weeding out incompetent physicians. You admit there are bad doctors but you also admit there is nothing you can do about it. Therefore, your peer review committees are a farce."

It was due to the failure of a peer review committee and a resultant newspaper article that the West Coast Editor of Medical Economics magazine (circulation: 500,000) first heard of me. I was interviewed and the article was published in the magazine in the fall of 1984. A readership survey showed that the article was the best-read item in that issue. The survey also revealed that most of the doctors, medical lawyers, and other health professionals who responded were overwhelmingly in favor of my program. I received telephone calls and letters from physicians throughout the United States. Some physicians even traveled great distances to meet with me and share their concerns and offer their support. Several of the doctors who contacted me donated books to my library, which is now believed to be the largest medical library owned by a lay organization in the United States.

Our organization's other activities have been equally successful. The Greeting Card Project has sent thousands of letters and cards to friends and relatives of convalescent home residents. The idea has been taken into other communities and several states.

The Emergency Loan Fund has assisted twenty-seven families who have become financially destitute because of a terminal or chronic illness and the accompanying high medical costs. On several occasions the fund has been responsible for preventing the loss of a family home.

In April, 1984, Consumers for Medical Quality, Incorporated drafted five proposals that would most definitely alter the way in which medicine is practiced in our state. These five proposals have received the endorsement of major labor unions and thousands of individuals. They are:

1. Require licensing re-examinations for physicians every five years.

Professional airline pilots are checked yearly and operators of trucks, buses, and other vehicles are routinely re-examined. Any failure or lessening of their expertise in the practice of their profession is deemed inherently dangerous to the public, yet, physicians, whose lack or diminution of skill or capacity is potentially more dangerous to a greater portion of the public, are never re-checked to determine their continued proficiency.

Thus, it is the duty and responsibility of the state in the exercise of its police powers to provide for the periodic re-examination of physicians practicing in the state to provide the continuing standard of medical care necessary to protect and promote the safety of the people.

2. Set the licensing fee in direct relation to the risk factor due to the physician's incompetence.

In all fairness to the many competent physicians, incompetent or impaired doctors should be required to pay a higher licensing fee, or an assessment, in the nature of a fine, to cover the heavy costs of added supervision and investigation.

3. Allow medical consumers the right of access to information regarding meritorious complaints filed against physicians.

Such information is necessary to enable a medical consumer to make an informed choice of physicians. In these days of multiplying malpractice suits, the medical community is increasingly shifting the responsibility for medical care to the patient-consumer.

The serious nature of the right of access to meritorious complaints is evidenced by many examples, i.e.: one physician, called a menace by the state Medical Standards Board, has been sued eight times for malpractice; has been before the state's licensing board for stripping a femoral artery instead of a vein during varicose vein surgery, causing the amputation of the patient's leg; has recently misdiagnosed an infection as wide-spread cancer, and caused the patient to undergo unnecessary surgery and to be hospitalized for six weeks; and is currently named in a three-million-dollar wrongful death suit. The list goes on and on.

4. Allow medical consumers the right of access to hospital mortality and morbidity rates.

The quality of medical care hospitals provide can vary dramatically. One hospital has a mortality rate of 50% while another nearby, similar-sized hospital has a 2-5% mortality rate.

Without mortality rate information, the medical consumer cannot make an informed decision as to which hospitals to avoid and which to patronize.

5. Allow medical consumers the right of access to the information regarding impaired physicians.

The state has a list of physicians on drug and alcohol rehabilitation programs. In order to be informed, the medical consumers need access to this list. According to one source, ". . . the average doctor will remain in the program three to five years. It's the old AA maxim that it takes that long to get the brains unscrambled."

As *Life Wish* goes to press, I am happy to report that the Senior Legislature of our state has adopted these five proposals to be among the "top ten" priority items to be presented into the State Legislature by an overwhelming 34-1 vote. The next step will be to find an author for this five-point bill; already, three of our state legislators have expressed an interest in authoring this bill.

In addition, a seventeen-page brief has been filed with the state's Department of Consumer Affairs by CMQ, seeking a Writ of Mandate that would compel the Medical Standards Board to perform its duties properly. It is the position of CMQ that the protection of the rights of patient-consumers is a matter of highest priority. In light of the many Legislative Audits and complaints filed against the Board, we must ask: how many more audits outlining MSB's deficiencies and patient-consumer documentations regarding the Board's incompetence are needed before the Director of Consumer of Affairs will take appropriate steps to protect the medical welfare of the public? We hope by this brief to obtain an order mandating MSB to protect medical consumers immediately, and in strict compliance with the law.

To remain silent is to condone and approve the misdeeds of others. As human beings it is our responsibility to try and correct injustice whenever we see it.

After reading the following story written by Karl Menninger, M.D., in his book *Whatever Became of Sin?* I was convinced that I could not remain silent. I share this story with you:

Who is to Blame?

We turn, angrily seeking someone to blame.

Who started the wretched, interminable war? Who ruined our air and oceans? Who filled our beautiful rivers and lakes with filth? Who beggared our paupers? Who crushed our blacks? Who alienated our youth? Who corrupted our business morals, our politics, our judicial system? No one? Who is the evil designer against the welfare of man? Is no one to blame when so much is wrong?

There is a parable in Matthew about someone secretly sowing weeds in a wheat field while the master and his servants slept. The servants were all for quickly cutting the weeds out, but the master said that at harvest time one could more effectively separate the wheat from the tares.

A fragment of manuscript has been found (or imagined!) which carries on this parable, though slightly at variance with the old text. An approximate translation reads:

And then the servants counseled together saying, "It would be much better to pull out those weeds right now rather than wait, but we must obey the master even when he is wrong. In the meantime, let us look about for the enemy who would do this evil thing to our master, who is kind to everyone and doesn't deserve this treatment." So they quietly inquired and made search in all the region round about, but they could find no one.

But one of the servants came privately to the chief steward at night saying, "Sir, forgive me, but I can no longer bear to conceal my secret. I know the enemy who sowed the tares. I saw him do it."

At this the chief steward was astonished and full of anger. But before punishing him, he demanded of the servant why he had not come forward sooner.

"I dared not," cried the servant. "I scarcely dared to come and tell you this even now. I was awake the night the weeds were sown. I saw the man who did it; he walked past me, seemingly awake and yet asleep, and he did not appear to recognize me. But I recognized him."

"And who was he, indeed?" asked the chief steward in great excitement. "Tell me, so he can be punished."

The servant hung his head. Finally, in a low voice he replied. "It was the master himself."

And the two agreed to say nothing of this to any man.

Afterword

by Steve Carroll

I married Paula in 1954. She was undoubtedly the most shy and sensitive woman I had ever met. It is this sensitivity that has always made her aware of the hurts and needs of others.

As with many newly married couples, we were on a very strict budget. One day during those early years, when Paula returned home, she was unusually quiet. She finally mustered enough courage to explain to me that we would have to delay the purchase of a needed household item because she had given the money away to a needy family. The reasons she gave for making such a decision justified her action more than adequately. How could I argue?

Over the years, this sort of thing happened quite regularly. I accepted her philanthropic ventures as being the very reason why I loved her so. My standard comment was: "You're doing your angel work—I can't interfere." At times she would go a little farther than I would have wished, but I could never disagree with her motivations.

One winter I insisted that she purchase a new coat. She only wore it a few times and then I never saw it again. Before I had figured out the obvious answer, I asked her where it was. With typical nonchalance, she answered that she had given it away to a woman who had no coat.

Yes, this was my Paula. If she wasn't giving our money and her clothes away, she was rescuing stray or lost dogs and cats and finding the owners or new homes for the orphaned pets.

In the succeeding years we worked hard together to build up our business. Through the lean years I was not able to show her my appreciation for all her support and hard work. Then the time came that I could afford to buy her a gift—something very special—a beautiful watch. I told her there was something at the local jeweler's for her to see and if she liked it, it was hers. When I saw her later that afternoon I expected her to be wearing the watch. She wasn't. She told me how the jeweler had put it on her wrist, but said that though it was beautiful, it was too expensive, so she left the store without it. I told her that the decision was mine and I bought the watch and gave it to her. She has worn it with great pride ever since.

Beginning in 1977, our lives suddenly changed. Paula was not only confronted with a serious health problem, but she also fell victim to a rapid succession of medical incompetency. It is most certainly not my nature to stand idly by and watch the person I love being hurt and humiliated. She definitely didn't deserve the treatment she received.

Those were very difficult years for both of us. I learned a great deal from Paula as I witnessed how she quietly and determinedly sought the truth concerning her own medical treatment. Throughout, she consistently assured me that everything was going to be all right.

Her predictions have come to pass: everything *is* all right.

Appendix

STATE MEDICAL BOARDS

Where to file medical consumer complaints:

Alabama Medical Licensure Commission
P.O. Box 887
Montgomery, AL 36101   (205) 832-5051

Alaska Department of Commerce and Economic
Development State Medical Board
Pouch "D"
Juneau, AK 99811   (907) 465-2541

Arizona Board of Medical Examiners
5060 N. 19th Ave.
Phoenix, AZ 85015   (602) 255-3751

Arkansas Board of Medical Examiners
P.O. Box 102
Harrisburg, AR 72432   (501) 578-2677

California Board of Medical Quality Assurance
1430 Howe Ave.
Sacramento, CA 95825   (916) 920-6411

Colorado Board of Medical Examiners
1525 Sherman
Denver, CO 80203   (303) 866-3988

Connecticut Board of Medical Examiners
79 Elm St.
Hartford, CT 06115   (203) 677-7784

Delaware Board of Medical Practice
Margaret O'Neill Bldg.
Dover, DE 19901   (302) 736-4753

District of Columbia Occupational and
Professional Licensing Division
605 G St., N.W.
Washington, DC 20001   (202) 727-6033

Florida Board of Medical Examiners
130 N. Monroe St.
Tallahassee, FL 32301   (904) 488-0595

Georgia Composite State Board of Medical Examiners
166 Pryor St., S.W.
Atlanta, GA 30303   (404) 656-7067

Hawaii Board of Medical Examiners
P.O. Box 3469
Honolulu, HI 96801   (808) 943-3338

Idaho State Board of Medicine
700 W. State St.
Boise, ID 83720   (208) 334-2822

Illinois Department of Registration and Education
320 W. Washington St.
Springfield, IL 62786   (217) 785-0896

Indiana Medical Licensing Board
700 N. High School Rd.
Indianapolis, IN 46224   (317) 232-2960

Iowa State Board of Medical Examiners
Executive Hills West
1209 E. Court Ave.
Des Moines, IA 50319   (515) 281-5171

Kansas State Board of Healing Arts
503 Kansas Ave.
Topeka, KS 66603   (913) 296-7413

Kentucky Board of Medical Licensure
Ephraim McDowell Dr.
Louisville, KY 40205   (502) 456-2220

Louisiana State Board of Medical Examiners
830 Union St.
New Orleans, LA 70112   (504) 524-6763

Maine Board of Registration in Medicine
100 College Ave.
Waterville, ME 04901   (207) 873-2184

Maryland Board of Medical Examiners
201 W. Preston St.
Baltimore, MD 21201   (301) 383-2020

Massachusetts Board of Registration in Medicine
100 Cambridge
Boston, MA 02202   (617) 727-3076

Michigan Board of Medicine
661 W. Ottawa St.
Lansing, MI 48933   (517) 373-0680

Minnesota State Board of Medical Examiners
717 S.E. Delaware
Minneapolis, MN 55414   (612) 623-5534

Mississippi State Board of Medical Licensure
2688-D Insurance Center Dr.
Jackson, MS 39216   (601) 354-6645

Missouri State Board of Registration for the Healing Arts
P.O. Box 4
Jefferson City, MO 65102 (314) 751-2334

Montana Board of Medical Examiners
1424 9th Ave., Bldg. 4
Helena, MT 59620 (406) 444-4284

Nebraska Board of Medical Examiners
301 Centennial Mall, S.
Lincoln, NE 68509 (402) 471-2115

Nevada State Board of Medical Examiners
1281 Terminal
Reno, NV 89502 (702) 329-2559

New Hampshire Board of Registration in Medicine
Health and Welfare Bldg.,
Hazen Dr.
Concord, NH 03301 (603) 271-1110

New Jersey State Board of Medical Examiners
28 W. State St.
Trenton, NJ 08608 (609) 292-4843

New Mexico Board of Medical Examiners
210 E. Marcy St.
Santa Fe, NM 87501 (505) 827-9930

New York State Board for Medicine
Cultural Education Center
Empire State Plaza
Albany, NY 12230 (518) 474-3817

North Carolina Board of Medical Examiners
222 N. Person St.
Raleigh, NC 27601 (919) 833-5321

North Dakota State Board of Medical Examiners
418 E. Rosser Ave.
Bismarck, ND 58501   (701) 223-9485

Ohio State Medical Board
65 S. Front St.
Columbus, OH 43215   (614) 466-3938

Oklahoma State Board of Medical Examiners
3013 N.W. 59th St.
Oklahoma City, OK 73112   (405) 848-6841

Oregon State Board of Medical Examiners
317 S.W. Adler St.
Portland, OR 97204   (503) 248-3746

Pennsylvania State Board of Medical Education
and Licensure
P.O. Box 2649
Harrisburg, PA 17105   (717) 787-2381

Rhode Island Division of Professional Regulation
75 Davis St.
Providence, RI 02908   (401) 277-2827

South Carolina State Board of Medical Examiners
1315 Blanding St.
Columbia, SC 29201   (803) 758-3361

South Dakota State Board of Medical and
Osteopathic Examiners
608 West Ave., N.
Sioux Falls, SD 57104   (605) 336-1965

Tennessee Board of Medical Examiners
R.S. Gass Station Office Bldg.
Nashville, TN 37216   (615) 741-7280

Texas Board of Medical Examiners
P.O. Box 13562 Capitol Station
Austin, TX 78711   (512) 473-9599

Utah Department of Registration
State Office
Salt Lake City, UT 84114   (801) 530-6003

Vermont Board of Medical Practice
109 State St.
Montpelier, VT 05602   (802) 828-2363

Virginia State Board of Medicine
517 W. Grace St.
Richmond, VA 23230   (703) 786-0575

Washington State Medical Boards
Division of Professional Licensing
P.O. Box 9649
Olympia, WA 98504   (206) 753-2205

West Virginia Board of Medicine
3412 - B Chesterfield Ave.
Charleston, WV 25304   (304) 348-2921

Wisconsin Medical Examining Board
P.O. Box 8936
Madison, WI 53708   (608) 266-2811

Wyoming Board of Medical Examiners
Hathaway Bldg.
Cheyenne, WY 82002   (307) 777-6463

Additional copies of *Life Wish* may be ordered by sending this card to:

Medical Consumers Publishing Company
2515 Santa Clara Avenue, #103
Alameda, CA 94501

Name _____

Address _____

City State Zip _____

Please send _____ copies of *Life Wish* @ $9.95 plus $2.00 shipping and handling (CA residents add $.60 (BART $.65) sales tax per book). Make check payable to: Medical Consumers Publishing Company.

- -

Additional copies of *Life Wish* may be ordered by sending this card to:

Medical Consumers Publishing Company
2515 Santa Clara Avenue, #103
Alameda, CA 94501

Name _____

Address _____

City State Zip _____

Please send _____ copies of *Life Wish* @ $9.95 plus $2.00 shipping and handling (CA residents add $.60 (BART $.65) sales tax per book). Make check payable to: Medical Consumers Publishing Company.